DYSLEXIA:
FROM THEORY TO INTERVENTION

NEUROPSYCHOLOGY AND COGNITION

VOLUME 18

The purpose of the Neuropsychology and Cognition series is to bring out volumes that promote understanding in topics relating brain and behavior. It is intended for use by both clinicians and research scientists in the fields of neuropsychology, cognitive psychology, psycholinguistics, speech and hearing, as well as education. Examples of topics to be covered in the series would relate to memory, language acquisition and breakdown, reading, attention, developing and aging brain. By addressing the theoretical, empirical, and applied aspects of brain-behavior relationships, this series will try to present the information in the fields of neuropsychology and cognition in a coherent manner.

The titles published in this series are listed at the end of this volume.

DYSLEXIA: FROM THEORY TO INTERVENTION

by

TORLEIV HØIEN

Dyslexia Research Foundation,
Stavanger, Norway

and

INGVAR LUNDBERG

Department of Psychology,
Göteborg University, Sweden

KLUWER ACADEMIC PUBLISHERS

DORDRECHT / BOSTON / LONDON

Library of Congress Cataloging-in-Publication Data.

ISBN 0-7923-6309-4

Published by Kluwer Academic Publishers,
P.O. Box 17, 3300 AA Dordrecht, The Netherlands.

Sold and distributed in North, Central and South America
by Kluwer Academic Publishers,
101 Philip Drive, Norwell, MA 02061, U.S.A.

In all other countries, sold and distributed
by Kluwer Academic Publishers,
P.O. Box 322, 3300 AH Dordrecht, The Netherlands.

This volume is a translation from Dysleksi: Fra Teori til Praksis
edited by T. Høien and I. Lundberg.
Published by Ad Notam Gyldendal, 1997

Printed on acid-free paper

Printed in the Netherlands.

TABLE OF CONTENTS

PREFACE

By the end of the 1980's dyslexia research had come of age in many countries, perhaps most particularly in the Nordic countries. Part of the impetus for the research was a growing need on the part of special teachers, school psychologists and others for solid, verified knowledge about reading and writing problems. In the decades leading up to the 1980's, it had become increasingly clear that individuals who couldn't efficiently deal with written language had an enormous handicap, because the demands society and the work market made on literacy had increased so greatly. The number of young people who continued in school past the obligatory years also increased dramatically, and this made the problem of dyslexia especially obvious. Our first book together on dyslexia, which was published in Norwegian in 1991, came to fill an important role. It was soon translated into Swedish and Danish, and it was used as a textbook at a great many colleges and universities throughout the Nordic countries.

But science rarely stands still. Since our book was published, a veritable tidalwave of new studies have been published in a growing number of journals or presented at international conferences. Our knowledge of dyslexia has expanded in breadth and depth the last ten years. The cross-disciplinary and multidisciplinary nature of reading research has become ever clearer. Neurobiology has made great advances in imaging techniques, allowing us to peer into the brains of living, thinking people. Molecular genetics is well on its way to demonstrating how a propensity for dyslexia is inherited. The fields of psychology and linguistics have increased our understanding of what language is and how children acquire and develop language skills, topics of direct relevance to the study of dyslexia. Better methods for diagnosing and remediating the condition have also been developed. In the field of education we see several new and promising approaches entailing early intervention and prevention in the pre-school years. Personal computers, perhaps the icon of the 1990's, are being increasingly often used for training reading and writing skills, and also to help compensate for the lack of those skills.

Because of a great many inquiries from scholars in many countries, we were persuaded to publish an English-language version of our book from 1997. The present book is, we hope, not merely a *translation* of our book, but a fairly thorough reworking of it with an eye to communicating with the international community of scholars. Dyslexia is not confined to any one language group. Any society with an alphabetical language (and that includes of course all the societies in Europe) will be marked by the condition. The problems dyslexic children in Finland, Greece, or the U.S. have are fundamentally the same, even though there may be some variation in how they are expressed, due to variation in the regularity of spelling in the languages in question. But fundamentally the problems and the condition are the same. Therefore, good research conducted in, say, Denmark, is immediately relevant to conditions in the U.S. or Great Britain. But, sadly, much good Scandinavian research has not been readily available to scholars who are unfamiliar with these languages.

Not only has our knowledge of dyslexia gained in breadth and depth the last ten years or so; it has to a certain measure also acquired an additional focus. Sociologists and others have contributed studies of the societal conditions that create and maintain the handicap, and the social constructions which constitute a concept like dyslexia. New perspectives on knowledge, teachers, and pupils have come to the fore, and at the same time we find a growing interest in qualitative methods in the behavioural sciences. Among other things, these qualitative methods grant us a more complete view of the disorder, by allowing dyslexics to tell us about their experiences. To a certain degree we have tried to reflect these new perspectives in the present book, and we acknowledge the value a social view of dyslexia can provide, in addition to the traditional medical and individual-oriented perspective.

The rapid pace of scientific advancement, and the pace of social change in general, provide ample reason for a new book about an old problem. Of course, while we have tried to provide a fairly complete picture of the status of our knowledge and theories today, we know full well that it is impossible to present in a single volume more than a selection of facts and theories. We have tried to eschew the trendy theories that come and go and the undocumented factoids that play well in the media, and we have tried instead to focus on research results that would seem to have a long shelf-life and that have been verified in many different studies.

Research in the last decade has provided more and more support for the hypothesis that (1) dyslexia is first and foremost a problem in decoding written words, or a problem in quickly and accurately identifying written words, and (2) that this problem is rooted in a deficit in the pupil's phonological system (his/her ability to deal with language-sounds). Because this view has been confirmed in a great many studies, it forms the backbone of the present book. But we are nonetheless open for other explanations of reading problems, such as general problems in automaticity and problems in recognizing visual patterns. Both of these alternative explanations are treated in this book. But the theoretical model we have based much of our work on grants special status to the reader's phonological system. (This model, incidentally, is virtually the same as the model we first presented in our book in 1991.)

There is nothing more practical than a good theory, as an old saying would have it. We believe that the myriad of practical problems encountered in diagnosing and treating reading problems become easier to deal with when you have a deep, theoretical understanding of the condition and its etiology. Nevertheless, no child has ever been helped by the teacher's *theory* alone. True learning can only take place in an environment imbued with mutual respect.

Preface comes first, but is written last, thus giving us the chance to express our indebtedness to our many friends, colleagues, and students who through the years have provided us with so many constructive criticisms and shared so many insights with us. To them all: thank you. In particular we would like to thank our secretary, Jette Marie Harbo, whose patience and editorial talent we have profited greatly from. We are also greatly indebted to our translators, Michael Evans (chapters 1-4) and Susan Schanche (chapters 5-8). Michael Evans also served as our chief translator and adaptor, to whom we owe many of the English spelling and phonological examples in the early chapters.

Stavanger, Norway, January 2000

Torleiv Høien and Ingvar Lundberg

CHAPTER 1

WHAT IS DYSLEXIA?

Anyone who visits a classroom will notice striking differences among the students, both physical and mental differences, despite the fact that the students are all the same age. Differences in temperament, motor skills, drawing skills, interests, reading ability, self-confidence, mathematics ability, verbal skills, and the like, are clearly evident. It is no easy task for a teacher to devise lessons that will accommodate every student in a given class.

Instruction in reading and writing is one of a school's most important responsibilities. Students' previous experience with language and books can differ as greatly as their background and abilities in other areas. But reading is a special subject; students who fail in learning to read will have a hard time in school, because so much of what they will have to learn in other subjects will depend on their reading and writing ability. Sometimes we as parents or teachers can be surprised by how difficult it is for some children to learn to read and write, even though they are alert, intelligent, and eager to learn. And sometimes we even hear about highly successful people who started out with significant reading and writing difficulties, but who eventually overcame their deficit, for example Auguste Rodin, Hans Christian Andersen, and Nelson Rockefeller.

On the other hand, there are those who have little trouble learning to read initially, but who nonetheless are significantly handicapped in their reading ability. They can read all the words correctly, but they just don't seem to grasp the import of what they have read. It is apparent that the technical side of reading - decoding words - doesn't seem to be closely associated with general intellectual ability. It seems likely that children who have a great deal of difficulty in learning to read have a cognitive deficit that is sharply limited in scope.

In order to characterize children of normal (or high) intelligence who show significant reading and writing difficulties, terms such as *dyslexia, word blindness,* or *specific reading and writing deficit* have been put forth. In this book we will use the term *dyslexia*, even though we use the term somewhat differently than has been common. We use the term in part because it has come in to common parlance, because it is short, and because it possibly best describes what we are talking about - a difficulty with written words. The Greek prefix *dys* means difficult or hard, *lexia* refers to words. The term word-blind doesn't function as well for our purpose, as it seems to imply a vision problem. The term 'specific reading and writing difficulties' is accurate, but unwieldy.

We choose to use the term dyslexia when describing *significant and persistent* reading difficulties. We are aware that there are risks in using terms like these - regardless of which one you choose. For one thing, they sound 'official', thereby giving an aura of greater precision and insight than we actually have. Secondly, there is always the risk that a student who is given this kind of diagnosis will feel singled out and stigmatized for life. But on the other hand, it is all too obvious for both the failing student and his classmates that his problem is massive and won't go away despite all the remedial instruction he is getting. In fact, being labeled a dyslexic is comforting to many; the label indicates a specific functional failing and not an general intellectual weakness.

It is also important to note that some of the students who test poorly in reading in the first and second grades, go on to conquer their difficulties without extra initiatives by the school. In our terminology, these students are not dyslexic; they just need extra time to acquire reading skills. Other students, however, have reading difficulties that persist due to their dyslexic character (Bruck, 1992; 1998; Jacobson and Lundberg, forthcoming.) Therefore it is important that those who are responsible for diagnosing dyslexia are careful to avoid drawing hasty conclusions from the results of individual tests. Making a diagnosis of dyslexia is a dilemma: We don't want to label students as dyslexic when their difficulties are only temporary, yet still it is crucial that those students who really are in the danger zone get the help they need early in their education (Juel, 1996; Lundberg, 1994; Santa and Høien, 1999; Wasik and Slavin, 1993).

The first scientific reports on dyslexia among school students date from about 100 years ago. A German ophthalmologist was the first to use the term dyslexia (Berlin 1887). However, he used this term to describe the reading difficulty noted in some adult patients suffering from brain damage. The English pediatrician Morgan was the first to describe childhood dyslexia. He coined the term 'word-blindness' (Morgan, 1896). Among the early medical pioneers, we can also mention the Scottish ophthalmologist Hinshelwood (1917).

In America, Samuel Orton was the first great dyslexia researcher. In the 1920's he formulated a theory that the visual impression of the written word is stored in both the dominant hemisphere of the brain (the left in most cases), and in the non-dominant hemisphere (usually the right). In the non-dominant hemisphere, the written word is stored as a mirror image. He then theorized that reading difficulties arose when neither hemisphere clearly dominated the other. Unstable hemisphere dominance, he thought, would lead to letters and words being reversed. For example, the word "mad" could be perceived as "dam." Even though this part of Orton's theory ultimately proved false, many of his observations about dyslexia have been valuable to later researchers. In honor of Orton's pioneering efforts, the *Orton Dyslexia Society* was founded in 1949. This organization has been one of the foremost in the world when it comes to research and the organizing of international conferences. The organization has recently changed its name to *The International Dyslexia Society.*

Every once in a while the question is raised as to whether dyslexia really exists. A question like this can seem strange amid the common acceptance that the term dyslexia has gained. Nevertheless, one cannot ignore the fact that there are people who believe that dyslexia is merely a social construct, held up by special education teachers in order to promote their own interests. They believe that the difficulties that so-called dyslexics encounter are only cosmetic, and point to the fact that many so-called dyslexics have done very well in life despite their difficulties. We have to admit that the term dyslexia not particularly well defined. It is therefore important that one is willing to question and discuss the term's definition.

The Problem of Definition

Since dyslexia first gained the attention of the scientific community, the definition of the term itself has been a recurring problem. After much work and many compromises, the World Federation of Neurology agreed in 1968 on the following definition of dyslexia:

> A disorder manifested by the difficulty in learning to read, despite conventional instruction, adequate intelligence and sociocultural opportunity. It is dependent upon fundamental cognitive disabilities, which are frequently of constitutional origin.

As we can see, this definition doesn't speak to what characterizes dyslexia, beyond the difficulty in achieving normal reading ability. We get more information about what dyslexia is *not*, and the definition is mainly concerned with the criteria for exclusion. Dyslexia then becomes all the reading difficulties that cannot be explained.

One of the main problems with the traditional definition is that it is tied to the general intellectual level of the person; dyslexia is the condition we have when there is a clear discrepancy between the person's reading ability and other intellectual ability. As we noted above, we are surprised when we see the great difficulties some bright students have in acquiring reading ability; we naturally expect that intelligent pupils will easily learn to read, and we imagine that confident reading is one of the many signs of high intelligence. So when we observe an exception to this rule, we are surprised and take note of it. But in fact it appears that the first reading skill that pupils learn, how to decode words, depends very little on the pupil's level of general intelligence. Summarizing the results of many investigations of the correlation between intelligence and reading ability in the first school years, we find a correlation that is on average only +0.30 to +0.40. This means that only 10 to 15 percent of the variation in reading ability we see among students can be explained by the variation in their general intellectual ability. We should therefore expect to find all levels of intelligence present among the poorest readers. So when some of the studies of poor readers show a significant overrepresentation of students of lower intelligence, this should be attributed in part to the fact that many intelligence tests (for example WISC-R) include tasks that are especially difficult for poor readers – e.g. vocabulary tests (Siegel, 1992; Stanovich, 1991).

There is therefore good reason to question the wisdom of the so-called discrepancy definition. For more a more comprehensive discussion on the relationship between intelligence and dyslexia, see the special issue of *Dyslexia*, volume 2, 1997; Aaron (1997); Lyon (1995) and Reid (1995).

The popularity of discrepancy-based definitions can most likely be ascribed to the attention given to a handful of well-known, highly gifted people with dyslexia. However, there is no scientific basis for assuming that people of low intelligence cannot have dyslexia (Siegel, 1992). Still, we find that the discrepancy between intellectual and reading abilities is used as a criterion for diagnosis of dyslexia in both *Diagnostic and Statistical Manual of Medical Disorder – IV*(DSM-IV) (American Psychiatric Association, 1994) and in *ICD-10 Classification of Mental and Behavioural Disorders* (ICD-10) (World Health Organization, 1993). One possible reason for wishing to keep a discrepancy criterion in the definition could be the laudable inclination to avoid that dyslexic students of normal intellectual abilities will be perceived as dumb.

Are there any special symptoms that characterize dyslexia? Writing about dyslexia would certainly be much easier if the disorder were a sharply delimited disorder, one that you either have or you don't have. In medicine this is very often the case: The child either has chicken-pox or she doesn't. But this just isn't the case with dyslexia. The line separating dyslexics from all the other people who don't read particularly well is not at all clear-cut. Dyslexia may be likened to obesity. Everyone recognizes a really obese person. But at what point does 'somewhat overweight' become 'true obesity'? The exact line between the two is arbitrary and varies from culture to culture. Similarly fluid boundaries are found in a host of other school subjects. Which children are exceptionally gifted (or hopelessly untalented) in music, or the visual arts, or in sports? It all depends on where we wish to put the dividing line. However, unlike these other subjects, poor reading ability can have devastating consequences. Society demands competency in reading and writing in ways it does not demand a base-level ability in drawing, singing, or playing football.

Dyslexia, then, involves a difficulty in attaining normal reading ability. Where we set the boundary for dyslexia will necessarily be somewhat arbitrary. Among other things, it will depend on what level of reading ability we deem necessary for a person to function in society. Those who cannot reach the prescribed level, despite hard work and proper instruction, will be deemed dyslexic. Merely stating this, however, isn't of much help. Strictly speaking, our definition only says that people with major reading problems are dyslexic.

If dyslexia is a more basic condition, a circumscribed weakness of a linguistic module with a neurobiological and genetic cause, we should be careful with referring to the manifest reading achievement. At least in principle, one can conceive of dyslexic individuals with adequate reading skills as a result of successful compensation. However, their basic linguistic weakness may still be there and can be revealed in stressful tasks normally not met in everyday life.

Reading is both Decoding and Comprehension

Perhaps we can come a step closer to an understanding of dyslexia by examining what reading is. Somewhat simplified, we can differentiate between two components: decoding and comprehension. Decoding is the technical side of reading: seeing a string of letters and knowing that they represent, say, the word *nation.* Decoding involves the ability to exploit the alphabetical principle, or code, in order to decipher written words. This component involves both laborious and time-consuming processes (such as sounding out letters and syllables) and the instantaneous, automatic word recognition that characterizes the good reader. The comprehension component, for its part, requires more in the way of cognitive resources. Comprehending a text includes such processes as connecting the text to one's own experiences and frames of reference, drawing conclusions from the text, formulating interpretations of it, and the like. This kind of thought process is, in principle, the same kind of process that one engages in when listening to another person read aloud.

The fact that decoding and comprehension are two separate processes becomes apparent when we look at various everyday situations. Sometimes, in the midst of reading aloud for a child, we 'come to' and discover that we have no idea what we've been reading. We've been fluidly decoding the words, but our conscious thoughts were off on a tangent. As long as we keep reading off the words, the child oftentimes doesn't notice that our thoughts have wandered. Or other times we'll be reading a book or newspaper when we suddenly wake up and discover that absolutely nothing on the page has 'sunk in'. Our eyes have followed the words on the page from left to right, line after line, yet no comprehension has taken place.

Extensive research has shown that the primary problem with dyslexia can be identified as a deficit in the decoding process (for overview, see Adams, 1990). Dyslexic readers' problems with comprehension can be seen, in general, as a secondary problem. Comprehension problems for these pupils are mainly a result of poor word-decoding ability.

An important question in connection with the definition of dyslexia is which criteria should be used as a basis for classification of word decoding difficulties (Berninger and Abbot, 1994; Fletcher and Foorman, 1994). As we have mentioned, there is no clear, unanimously accepted measure for the boundary between the lower limit of 'less than good' reading and the degree of poor reading we wish to term dyslexia. Students' ability to decode words, as measured with a good test of word-decoding, are distributed along the familiar bell curve. What percentage of students are 'poor readers' depends simply on where one draws the dividing line. If one chooses to set the boundary at -1 standard deviation (SD) below the mean, then statistically 16 percent of the students will be classified as 'poor readers' (see Figure 1.1).

If we instead choose to set -2 SD as our cut-off point, the percentage will fall dramatically to about 2 percent (Figure 1.1). In the literature we often see different researchers operating with various numbers as to the percentage of children with reading problems. These percentages vary from 1 percent to 20 percent. In the main this is the result of their using different cut-off points in their definitions. But another factor which leads to these differing results is that the various researchers often use tests which are actually testing different skills. Some of the tests emphasize almost exclusively the ability to decode individual words or nonwords (experimentally devised 'words' such as *spim* or *merts*), while other tests in addition seek to measure the student's ability to comprehend various genres of texts.

We propose that a necessary criterion of dyslexia is serious and persistent difficulty in decoding words. Decoding ability must be measured with a well-accepted, standardized decoding test. Somewhat arbitrarily we can set our cut-off point at the tenth percentile (i.e. the lowest-scoring 10 percent). Before labeling a student as dyslexic, one should give him or her other decoding tests as well. In our

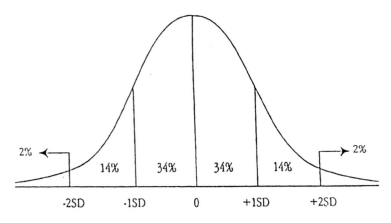

Figure 1.1. The normal distribution of students' decoding ability. SD = standard deviation.

opinion the diagnosis dyslexia should be based on a broad evaluation of a student's decoding ability. In most cases, a student's decoding difficulties will be accompanied by serious writing difficulties (Moats, 1995).

The dyslexic student is unable to develop the reliable, automatic decoding ability that is the hallmark of the good reader. Reading, for the dyslexic student, is like riding a bicycle against the wind: strenuous, frustrating, and no fun. So we shouldn't be surprised that so many dyslexics give up. Reading for them entails such a great mental effort and yields so little in return that it doesn't seem worth the bother. This puts them at risk for winding up in a very vicious circle: Achieving automatic word recognition requires practice - that is, many encounters with the written word. Dyslexics shun reading because they read poorly, so they don't get the practice that is required to obtain solid decoding skills (cf. The Matthew Effect, Stanovich, 1986).

A New American Working Definition

In 1994, the Orton Dyslexia Society Research Committee, in cooperation with the leaders of the National Center for Learning Disabilities and researchers from the National Institute of Child Health and Human Development, developed a new working definition for dyslexia (The Orton Dyslexia Society Research Committee, April, 1994). We will see that this definition has many similarities to our definition (Høien and Lundberg, 1991). Here is the first part of the American definition of dyslexia:

> Dyslexia is one of several distinct learning disabilities. It is a
> specific, language-based disorder of constitutional origin
> characterized by difficulties in single word decoding, usually
> reflecting insufficient phonological abilities.

This new definition stresses that the main characteristic of dyslexia is connected to word decoding, and that difficulties with decoding are due to a deficit in phonological abilities. (We treat phonological abilities in Chapter 4). Moreover, dyslexic difficulties are tied to the ability to read individual words.

This corresponds with extensive international research, which shows that good readers do not need to exploit the context in order to recognize a written word (for an overview, see Share and Stanovich, 1995). Good readers have developed well-functioning decoding skills, and automatic decoding is, as mentioned, a necessary prerequisite to understanding written material. When the young reader can automatically decode most of the words, then he or she can apply more cognitive resources to the comprehension process, a task which requires both attention and reflection. Readers who have great difficulties with decoding often use contextual information when decoding words in a text. This often results in much guessing and many errors.

According to this definition, dyslexic students' decoding problems are mainly caused by difficulties in phonological skills. This is in line with recent dyslexia research, which shows a connection between poor decoding ability and poor phonological ability (Brady and Shankweiler, 1991; Lundberg and Høien, 1997; Lundberg, Olofsson and Wall, 1980). Dyslexics score poorly on tests consisting of different types of phonological tasks. They have poorly defined conceptions of the sound structure of words, they have poor articulation and a weak phonological short-term memory. One often finds that dyslexics have difficulty remembering new words and names. They also have problems repeating back phonologically complex words or nonwords (Brady, 1997). Poor phonological short-term memory also has a negative influence on reading comprehension (Stothard and Hulme 1992). Here is the second part of the American definition of dyslexia:

> These difficulties in a single word decoding are often unexpected
> in relation to age and to other cognitive and academic abilities; they
> are not the result of generalized developmental disability or sensory
> impairment. Dyslexia is manifested by variable difficulty with
> different forms of language, often including, in addition to problems

with reading, a conspicuous problem with acquiring proficiency
in writing and spelling.

The definition still holds with the idea of discrepancy-based criteria, even though it
does not set exact demands as to the size of the discrepancy between reading ability
and other intellectual abilities; it merely states that the discrepancy is 'often
unexpected'.

Some researchers have found it useful to compare reading comprehension
with listening comprehension (see Aaron, 1989; Joshi, Williams, and Wood, 1998).
According to these researchers, dyslexics will score significantly lower when tested
for reading comprehension ability than when tested for how well they comprehend
texts that are read aloud to them. A discrepancy between these two scores would
indicate dyslexia. This approach, which seems reasonable at first glance, is actually
rather problematic, especially when applied to adolescents and adults. A person's
achievement in listening comprehension is determined mainly by his or her language
skills, and these skills are to a certain degree acquired through practice in reading
(see Oakhill et al., 1998; Juel, 1988). And if there is one thing that we know about
dyslexics, it is that they don't read a lot. Another problem with this approach is
finding texts that are substantially similar for the purpose of comparing reading and
listening comprehension.

The new American definition concludes by underlining the close
connection between dyslexia and language difficulty, and it claims that dyslexia is
an impediment to achieving good writing and spelling abilities (spelling includes
both accurate written representation of a word as well as oral spelling).

Our Definition of Dyslexia

Our definition of dyslexia is the same as we presented several years ago (Høien and
Lundberg, 1991):

> Dyslexia is a disturbance in certain language functions which
> are important for using the alphabetic principle in the decoding of
> language. The disturbance first appears as a difficulty in obtaining
> automatic word decoding in the reading process. The disturbance
> is also revealed in poor writing ability. The dyslexic disturbance is
> generally passed on in families and one can suppose that a genetic
> disposition underlies the condition. Another characteristic of dyslexia
> is that the disturbance is persistent. Even though reading ability can
> eventually reach an acceptable performance level, poor writing
> skills most often remain. With a more thorough testing of the
> phonological abilities, one finds that weakness in this area often
> persists into adulthood.

More simply, we define dyslexia as:

A persisting disturbance in the coding of written language, which
has its cause in a deficit in the phonological system.

As in the American definition, we have attempted to speak to what dyslexia is:
significant difficulty with word decoding and writing ability due to a failure of the
phonological system. For reasons outlined above, we do not wish to define the
disorder on the basis of discrepancies.

According to our definition, an individual can suffer from dyslexia
regardless of his or her general intellectual ability. It follows, then, that there are
highly gifted individuals with dyslexia, as well as individuals with lesser abilities
who have no problem in acquiring good decoding abilities. Students with low
intellectual abilities, sensory handicaps, or emotional disturbances can also have
dyslexia. Obviously, in such cases, the extra handicap will exacerbate reading
problems.

In Figure 1.2, we summarize our principle views on dyslexia. The *primary
symptoms* of dyslexia are problems with word decoding and spelling. We suppose
that the primary symptoms are the direct result of a *deficit in the phonological
system* (see Chapter 4). The decisive role that we assign to the phonological process
in word decoding does not exclude the possibility that there are other factors that can
create problems for dyslexics (Fletcher and Morris, 1997; Stanovich et al., 1997a,
1997b, 1997c). Various researchers have focused on possible connections between
dyslexia and a deficit in the ability to identify sequentially presented sensory
impressions, between dyslexia and difficulties with orthography (how words are
spelled), with semantics (what words mean), syntactics (how sentences are
constructed), and morphology (how words are built up of roots, prefixes and
suffixes). The problem with these approaches, however, is that it is difficult to
determine to what degree a deficit in one or more of these areas is merely a
consequence of the person's phonological problems, or whether these other kinds of
deficits are truly independent causes of the poor reading. This is a particularly
significant question when it comes to the relationship between phonology and
orthography. Despite the fact that these other areas are of great interest to reading
research, we have chosen to use the term dyslexia when describing cases in which
the decoding difficulties are brought about by phonological problems.

Behind this phonological disturbance, we can, in some instances, count on
finding abnormalities in neurological structure and function. Neurological
abnormalities can in turn be seen as the result of a complicated interplay between
genetic factors and environmental influences, an interplay that starts as early as
during fetal development (see Chapter 6).

We have looked at the chain of causes that underlie the primary symptoms.
We turn now to the *secondary symptoms*. We have already mentioned poor reading
comprehension. Problems with mathematics can also appear as a result of reading
difficulties. The poor self-image that is often observed among dyslexic students can
also be considered a secondary symptom. Similarly, socioemotional adjustment and
behavioral problems can develop as a result of dyslexia. Likewise, irregular eye
movements are also most likely a result of reading difficulty rather than the cause
(McConkie, 1983).

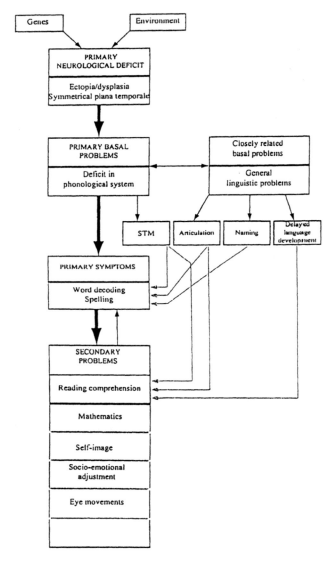

Figure 1.2. Primary components (symptoms and casual factors) of dyslexia.

Dyslexics have phonological problems, that is, a linguistic deficit in which at least one part of the language function is affected. It is therefore not surprising that many dyslexics have other linguistic problems as well. In these instances we speak of *closely related basal difficulties.* These can surface as short-term memory problems, difficulty with naming things, poor articulation, and delayed language development. These related basal difficulties can have a negative influence on the process of learning to read. Poor short-term memory makes it difficult to understand long sentences, or sentences with difficult syntax. Problems with naming can make it difficult for students to learn new words; this hinders the building of the good vocabulary that is needed for reading comprehension. Furthermore, difficulties with phonological discrimination and articulation hinder the young reader in learning the precise phonological identities of words; having only fuzzy knowledge of what a given word sounds like makes it well-nigh impossible for the reader to learn the word (Brady, 1997; Elbro, 1996).

There are other problems that can be associated with dyslexia, even though they may not appear as often as the 'closely related' basal problems. What we term the 'related' basal problems are such deficits as poor motor skills, attention problems, poor concentration, difficulty with sequences of information, etc. These related basal problems can also have a negative impact on word decoding.

There are also other symptoms which are neither secondary nor related, yet which are often regarded as characteristic of dyslexia. These symptoms include defects in one or more of the senses, or being left-handed. Controlled studies, however, have shown that these traits are merely *incidental symptoms.* They occur just as often among students with normal reading abilities and therefore do not shed any light on the nature of dyslexia. It is important, however, that we do not overlook the possibility that sensory and perceptual defects can be obstacles to good reading for individual students, even causing their reading difficulties, despite the fact that this does not fit our definition of dyslexia. In Chapter 7 we address recent research on how various obstructing mechanisms can impede the process of learning to read.

Subgroups of Dyslexia

One need not work long with dyslexics before noticing how differently they go about reading and writing. Some read slowly and cautiously, while others rush through a text at high speed, making many wild guesses along the way. An analysis of reading and writing errors reveals great individual variations in both numbers and types of errors. Analyses show clearly that dyslexics do not make up a homogeneous group. From a teaching point of view, of course, this creates problems. And it is therefore not surprising that researchers have often attempted to subdivide dyslexics into more homogeneous *subgroups.* The purpose of this kind of categorization is clear: If we can separate the students into reasonably homogeneous subgroups, we may be able to design more appropriate teaching methods to meet the specific needs of each of the subgroups (see Stanovich et al., 1997a, 1997b).

In dyslexia research it was not until about 1970 that the urge to subgroup dyslexics came to the fore. This interest is voiced in a number of articles on the theme, and these articles are characterized by a wide variety of goals and purposes. The original incentive for subgrouping was the need for more differentiated diagnosis and treatment. Later, the need for more precise research hypotheses and theories also came into the picture. The more theory-oriented interest in defining the term and phenomenon of dyslexia has revived the question as to whether there are distinct groups of reading difficulties which may be classified under the term dyslexia.

The spectrum of literature on subgrouping leaves a mottled impression. Categorizing and comparing the various contributions is no easy task; the terminology, goals and methods of the researchers are that disparate. The quality of the work and the conclusions derived from it vary considerably as well. One study, say a statistical analysis of scores on a series of tests, could yield (say) five reasonably well-defined subgroups of dyslexics. Here the various kinds score profiles would characterize the five subgroups. But with another method you could find a different number of subgroups entirely. More distressingly, two individuals who belong to the same subgroup when we apply one method may fall into two different subgroups when another classification approach is used. It is also obvious that the tests that are chosen to make up the battery will critically determine the result of subgroup classification (for an overview, see Lyon, 1994).

Empirical Research and the Subgrouping of Dyslexics

At the end of the 1960's, Johnson and Myklebust (1967) suggested a division between two types of dyslexia: *auditive dyslexia* and *visual dyslexia*. Auditive dyslexia, according to them, is characterized by a difficulty in discriminating between similar phonemes, and problems in linking phonemes together ('blending') when trying to read a word. Students with visual dyslexia, on the other hand, have difficulty understanding, interpreting and remembering letters and images of words. They have a tendency to confuse letters that are visually similar, and words that resemble each other.

Boder (1971, 1973) studied the reading and writing errors made by dyslexics. She envisioned that many of the linguistic and cognitive processes underlying reading and writing were common to both activities, or in some cases at least tightly interwoven. She believed, therefore, that in order to obtain a reasonably complete picture of how a student deals with written language, the analysis of the student's reading behavior would have to be supplemented by a similar analysis of his writing behavior. She undertook a qualitative analysis of both reading and writing errors, and on the basis of this analysis she suggested three subgroups: *dysphonetic dyslexia, dyseidetic dyslexia*, and *alexia*. Dysphonetic dyslexia, according to Boder, is caused primarily by a deficit in phonological ability which hinders the student in reading unfamiliar words or nonwords. Their attempts at spelling are characterized by many phonological errors; their spellings often could not be read off as the target word. Dyseidetic dyslexia, on the other hand, reflects a failure in the ability to perceive words as units. These children read phonetically by carefully sounding out the letters in each word. Their writing is phonologically acceptable, but they are often unable to spell correctly irregular words, that is, words that do not follow the most common spelling rules. Broder's alexia subgroup is made up of dyslexics who have deficits in both phonological and visual processing. (We should point out that Boder uses the term alexia in a way that differs from normal usage in reading research, where alexia usually refers to acquired reading difficulty due to a trauma to the brain, such as a stroke.) According to Boder, 67 percent of her dyslexics were dysphonetic, 10 percent were dyseidetic, and 23 percent were of the mixed alexic type.

Gjessing (1977) operated with a greater number of dyslexia subgroups: *auditive dyslexia, visual dyslexia, auditive/visual dyslexia, emotional dyslexia, instructional dyslexia,* and *other forms* of dyslexia.

Auditive dyslexia is characterized by great difficulties with the sounds of spoken language. Auditive dyslexics often show a retarded development of language skills. In both reading and writing they show symptoms of a deficit in aural discrimination and memorization abilities. They have problems discriminating between similar phonemes, especially those pairs of consonants which are distinguished by voicing (for example, *b-p, d-t, k-g,* and *v-f*). Another characteristic trait of the auditive dyslexic is a difficulty in sequencing and blending phonemes. Reading, for these students, often begins with guesses based on the word's general appearance. When they are required to read phonologically - to really deal with the strings of letters instead of just guessing - they read very slowly, backtracking a lot to repeat letter-sounds and syllables. Students with auditive dyslexia will have reading problems that appear already in the first months of first grade, if the teaching is based on some sort of 'phonics' type of approach.

Visual dyslexia, for Gjessing, is characterized by problems with whole word reading, which makes the reader dependent on a laborious sounding-out technique even when he has had extensive exposure to reading material. It seems nearly impossible for this subgroup of dyslexics to identify even the most common words as visual shapes. Their reading is often peppered with complete reversals (*mad-dam, tap-pat*), and they easily confuse words of similar appearance (*map-may*). A striking trait among visual dyslexics is their phonological writing: '*pencil*' becomes '*pensil*', and '*tough*' becomes '*tuf*'. Furthermore, silent letters are left out : '*what*' becomes '*wat*', and '*love*' becomes '*lov*' and so on.

Gjessing's third subgroup, the *auditive/visual* dyslexics, consists of students who have difficulties in both of these areas. But according to Gjessing their auditive problems are primary.

The three final subgroups of dyslexia that Gjessing has formulated are not cases we traditionally wish to term dyslexia. In these subgroups, the students' reading problems are only secondary; some other type of problem is primary. Gjessing's 'emotional dyslexics' are those students' whose reading problems are caused by emotional problems, his 'instructional dyslexics' are those who have been subjected to poor teaching. His final subgroup, 'other forms', is a grab bag of miscellaneous.

These initial attempts at defining subgroups of dyslexia were for the most part based on purely clinical data. These subgroups no doubt seemed to appear in the data; they were not formulated on the basis of explicit theoretical models of how we read and write. This is unfortunate, because a good model of reading and writing would be of great help when formulating various subgroups and when diagnosing individual students. The lack of theoretical foundation represents an obvious weakness in the early efforts at forming subgroups of dyslexia.

One problem with merely formulating subgroups on the basis of what you see in the data, instead of using an explicit model, is that we do not know the extent to which the observed discrepancies we are using to make the subgroups are merely a reflection of different environmental influences, for example instructional techniques. Reading is something that has to be taught and learned. Perhaps the 'auditive' or 'dysphonetic' dyslexics have simply not yet learned how to sound out words. This could well be the case if their teacher has emphasized whole-word reading at the expense of phonetically-based methods.

Or perhaps the different subgroups of dyslexia simply mirror different levels of reading development. Variations in reading ability due to age must be observed carefully. Older children normally have a larger repertoire of words that they can recognize on sight than younger children have. They have also learned more of the orthographic conventions used to represent words. For this reason, an older student reads not only better than a younger student, but *differently* as well.

When subgrouping is done primarily on the basis of the types of reading errors a student makes and the kinds of strategies he uses, there are several potential sources of error. For example, it is seldom easy to determine whether an error is visual or phonological. In order to classify an error as one or the other, the researcher has to be thoroughly familiar with the student's dialect, and this is often no easy matter. In many instances, errors that we first classify as phonological in nature can on the contrary be seen as evidence of a strong phonological capability. For example, an American student who writes the word *wash* as *warsch* may be making his 'mistake' because he has made an exceedingly fine phonological analysis of the sound of the word. Because we know that there is no letter *r* in *wash*, we may not be aware that some native speakers do in fact have an *r*-like sound in their pronunciation of the word. (More on this in Chapter 3.)

New hypotheses and new research methods can provide a sturdier basis for new ways of forming subgroups. An increasing understanding of the anatomy of the brain and its function will certainly have an effect on our future understanding of the causes, the symptoms, and the subgroups of dyslexia. Advances in molecular genetics may similarly contribute to further specification of subgroups.

From Subgrouping to Diagnosing, Based on a Model of Reading

In the 1970's it became common to form subgroups of *alexia* on the basis of a theoretical model on the word-recognition process (Marshall and Newcombe 1973). Alexia is the term we use for those reading difficulties which appear among previously good readers who have incurred brain damage. Most alexia patients are have had strokes.

The most commonly used model in alexia research was the so-called dual-route model. The dual-route model posits that there are two different strategies or 'routes' that normal readers can use to recognize a written word. One is the phonological strategy, by which the reader recodes letters and other sub-word units such as common letter-clusters (*br*, *-ough*, etc.) and syllables. This is often called 'sounding out' the word. The other strategy is the orthographic strategy. By means of the orthographical route we recognize the word in one fell swoop, as a unit. This is also called whole-word reading. (Both of these routes are treated more fully in the next chapter.)

On the basis of the dual-route model, researchers proposed several different ways to subgroup the various cases of alexia they were seeing. These subgroupings were based on the types of errors the individual reader committed, and his or her scores on test batteries. Unsurprisingly, given the reading model they were using, the two most central subgroups were *phonological alexia* (difficulties in using the phonological strategy) and *orthographic alexia*, sometimes termed 'surface dyslexia' (difficulties with the orthographic strategy).

In the beginning of the 1980's, researchers began to present various systems of subgrouping of *developmental dyslexia* that were based on the same model that was used for *alexia* (Coltheart et al., 1980). Much of this research was often based on case studies, and a common objection to it was that no control group of normal readers was used in the research.

Addressing this problem, Castle and Coltheart (1993) carried out a study using a group of dyslexics and an age-matched control group of normal readers. Students were asked to read aloud very irregular words; i.e. words with spellings so non-phonetical that it is difficult to sound them out. By and large, the student either recognizes these words or he doesn't, and this task is therefore thought to measure the efficacy of the reader's orthographic route. In order to measure how well their phonological route functioned, the students were asked to read aloud phonologically plausible nonwords, that is, pseudo-words like *spim* or *wug*. Because the child hasn't seen these 'words' before, we can be sure that when he reads them off with the desired pronunciation that he has sounded them out, i.e. used the phonological route. When Castle and Coltheart analyzed their data, they found support for three subgroups of dyslexia: *phonological dyslexia*, *orthographic dyslexia*, and *phonological/orthographic dyslexia*

An objection that can be raised to Castle and Coltheart's work is that their control group was age-matched, not matched for level of reading ability. In a more recent study by Manis et al. (1996) a replication of the Castle and Coltheart's study was done with a reading level-matched control group as well as an age-matched group. When the results from the reading level-matched controls were used as the criteria for defining poor and acceptable phonological and orthographic reading abilities, only one of the students in the group could be classified as an orthographic dyslexic. The main problem for the majority of test-group students was the phonological deficit. (We return to the need for a reading-level matched control group in the next section; in addition, see Bryant and Impey, 1986.)

Stanovich et al. (1997c) carried out a study of third-grade dyslexic students and first and second-grade students whose reading levels matched the dyslexic students'. In addition to tests that measured the ability to read irregular words and nonwords, they also used tests that mapped various phonological and orthographic subskills. This study shows that the main characteristic of all the dyslexics is a poorly developed, deficient phonological ability. The degree of phonological weakness varied among the dyslexics. According to Stanovich and his colleagues, orthographic dyslexia and phonological dyslexia can be explained as the product of just two factors: the severity of the child's phonological deficit, and the amount of the child's of exposure to print. On the basis of this assumption, orthographic dyslexia can be explained as the result of a milder form of phonological deficit combined with inadequate reading experience. Phonological dyslexia is then explained as being caused by a serious phonological deficit combined with normally sufficient exposure to print. An interesting question arises here: is it possible that some dyslexics have both good phonological abilities and adequate exposure to print, but nonetheless are unable to read orthographically? Recent research (Olson et al., 1997) seems to support this assumption.

On several occasions, we have suggested a 'process-analytical' approach to the diagnosing of dyslexia (Bjaalid and Høien, 1996; Høien and Legaard, 1991; Høien and Lundberg, 1989; Høien et al., 1989a; Legaard, 1987; Lundberg and Høien, 1990). A process-analytical approach is, as the term indicates, an approach based on an analysis of the individual reader's many word decoding subprocesses. Reading is a complex activity, and to understand why it sometimes goes wrong, we have to know about the processes that make it up. Our process-analytical approach is based on an explicit theory of how normal reading takes place. When diagnosing a poor reader, we give the student a number of tests which are designed to measure how well the various subprocesses function. These tests yield a profile of the individual reader's abilities. This profile takes into account both quantitative and qualitative factors inherent in the student's pattern of reading. The process analysis focuses not only on the student's weaknesses (reading and writing errors), but provides useful information about what he or she masters. This gives us a good basis for tailoring the remedial programme to the individual student. A process-analytical diagnosis is rooted in a theoretical model of the various strategies and subprocesses that normal word decoding is made up of. In the next chapter we will look closer at the word decoding process. But first we will address some of the different research methods that have been utilized in the study of dyslexia.

Methods in Dyslexia Research

Case studies

The 'classic' way of studying dyslexia as been through case studies - a legacy from the early studies of alexia. By looking closely at individuals with pronounced reading problems we are able to get a rich, detailed picture of the complex disorder as it manifests itself in an individual. As long as the researcher is guided by a scientific theory in his or her collection of data, case studies can yield invaluable information.

But the problem with case studies is that they are difficult to make generalizations from. You study an individual in depth; you find something interesting in his reading pattern; you form a theory as to what is going on. Now, how do you know if your new insight is relevant to any other reader on the face of the earth? When working with case studies, we don't know if we are seeing a unique, idiosyncratic pattern of symptoms, or if a lot of other readers, both good and poor, share this pattern. This is why case studies need to be augmented with other methods.

Comparing dyslexics with age-matched normal readers

Perhaps the most common research method involves selecting a group of dyslexics, usually on the basis of either exclusionary criteria or the discrepancy-based definition. A control group is then selected that matches the dyslexic group in all relevant aspects, typically including age, gender, classroom environment, intelligence, and social background. The idea is to form a control group that is just like the study group, except that they read normally. The researcher then gives both groups the same battery of tests. On some of the tests, pronounced differences between the groups turn up, for example in the realms of language function, short-term memory, eye-movement patterns, self-concept, etc. Where the differences between the groups are most obvious, one may think one has found some of the hallmarks of dyslexia, perhaps even the underlying causes of the disorder.

Still, one must be cautious. A difference that is observed between the two groups cannot simply be assumed to represent a causal factor, because that difference may in turn be caused by some other, more underlying factor. For example, when you compare a group of dyslexics with an age-matched control group, the dyslexics not only have poorer reading skills, but far less reading *experience* as well. Already by the time children are in the second grade, good readers read far more both in school and during their free time, than poor readers do. So some of the difference in scores on the test battery are most likely due to differences in the reading experience of the two groups, rather than a result of the difference in their reading abilities.

In an attempt to get around these kinds of interpretation problems, researchers in recent years have begun to use a different kind of control group. Instead of matching by age, it is becoming common to match the control group by *level of reading ability*. This generally means finding children who are a year or two younger than the study group. The point is that they are normal readers for their own age group.

Matching by reading level

By using a control group that reads on the same level as the dyslexics, it is easier to determine the causal factors. On can assume that the study group and the controls have approximately the same reading habits, in as much as they both struggle equally with texts. If the tests then show, for example, that the dyslexics have more difficulties in performing phonological tasks (e.g. segmenting phonemes, reading nonwords, reversing the order of syllables, etc.), despite being older than the control group, there is reason to believe that one has found a causal factor of dyslexia.

However, if the dyslexic group completes the tasks in the same way and at the same achievement level as the younger students in the control group, then we've found out nothing about causes.

Reading level comparisons were very popular in the 1980's (Vellutino and Scanlon, 1989). However, more recent research shows that this method is not without its statistical and methodological problems (Stanovich and Siegel 1994). Among other things, this method doesn't take into account all of the areas of variation in reading in the same way that, for example, sophisticated statistical analyses do.

Longitudinal studies

Some of the most informative studies we have are the longitudinal studies, where researchers have followed a group of children over an extended period of time, usually several years. This allows us to trace the development of the group, which grants us unique insight into the nature of dyslexia. One can, for example, measure specific functions early, even before reading instruction has begun, and find out how well a child's score predicts his or her later development. In the next chapter and in Chapter 4, we will look more closely and how longitudinal studies have helped us to better understand dyslexia. By following individuals over a period of time, we can also see whether dyslexia is reading development that is just a lot slower than normal, or whether the dyslexics read in a qualitatively different way, perhaps by finding ways of compensating for their deficit.

In recent years, sophisticated methods of statistical analysis of reading development have come into use (Francis et al., 1994). If we measure a group of young readers three or more times over the course of, say, two years, we can construct a mathematical curve that characterizes the course of development for each individual in the group. Then we can analyze the degree to which various factors (e.g. gender, socio-economic level, intelligence, motor skill development, etc.) can explain variation of the coefficient of the developmental curve. This kind of analysis, termed *multiple regression analysis,* gives us answers to some important questions: What are the factors that determine why some students make good progress in learning to read, while others take so much longer? A corresponding follow-up of individual students will also provide information about any stagnation in their reading development. Knowledge of this kind will be especially helpful in the work of diagnosing (Jacobson and Lundberg, in print).

Experimental studies

Strictly speaking, researchers cannot pinpoint causal factors without having an experimental plan in which the researcher experimentally varies just one variable or at most very few variables, while keeping the other factors constant or under control. Experiments like these, which are common in the natural sciences, allow the researcher to measure the extent that a change in one element causes a change in the function being studied. Purely experimental studies are very uncommon in dyslexia research; in fact, they are perhaps impossible. In a later chapter, we will see examples of training studies that approach this experimental ideal. These studies are only possible when the researchers make relatively firm inferences about causes and effects in phonological skills and reading development.

Recent techniques

Research methods in the biologically-oriented dyslexia research are developing rapidly. New methods for studying the brain's structure and function in living, conscious humans are also being developed. MRI (Magnetic Resonance Imaging) is perhaps one of the most promising techniques when it comes to the mapping of structural abnormalities in the brain (for a summary, see Hynd and Hiémenz, 1997). At the moment, functional MRI's (fMRI) are at the forefront of research. These give us the opportunity to study activity in the brain during the performance of various linguistic and cognitive tasks. Furthermore, there are incredible advances being made in the field of genetics. It is now possible to localize the genes that control development of several physical and psychological functions (Cardon et al., 1994). We will return to these techniques in Chapter 6.

Brief Summary

Reading involves two sub-tasks: decoding and comprehension. Serious decoding and spelling difficulties characterize dyslexia. Most often, the definition of dyslexia is rooted in exclusionary criteria: Dyslexia is what you have when all the other known factors are ruled out. This negative method for defining dyslexia does not shed much light on the causes of dyslexia. We have chosen to define the condition positively: *Dyslexia is a persisting disturbance in the coding of written language, which has its cause in a deficit in the phonological system.* At the same time, we are open to the possibility that there can be forms of dyslexia that are caused by a primary visual (orthographic) difficulty. By using this definition of dyslexia, we find dyslexics at all levels of intelligence and with additional, varying forms of emotional, educational, motivational, or physical handicaps.

Much attention has also been given to the efforts made in finding reliable methods for classifying dyslexia into well-defined subgroups. Researchers have mainly looked at three subgroups: auditive (phonological) dyslexia, visual (orthographic) dyslexia, and auditive-visual dyslexia. The purpose behind subgrouping has been to arrive at a more homogeneous subgroups of dyslexics. However, there are still large, individual differences among dyslexics within the subgroups. If one were to take into account all these individual differences, most likely the number of subgroups would need to be substantially increased. One alternative procedure for the diagnosing of dyslexia is to map the student's decoding abilities with the help of a model of normal reading. This method, also called process-analytical diagnosing, provides important information about the individual student's abilities in regard to the central subskills involved in decoding words.

In the study of dyslexia, researchers employed many different methods: case studies, comparisons between dyslexics and normal readers, reading level matching, longitudinal studies, and experimental studies. Having many different types of approaches is useful when it comes to gaining comprehensive knowledge about the problem of dyslexia.

CHAPTER 2

DECODING DIFFICULTIES - A MAJOR SYMPTOM OF DYSLEXIA

Reading ability is a complex skill that builds on a number of decoding and comprehension processes. *Decoding* allows the reader to recognize and pronounce the word, and thereby access its meaning. This skill takes time to build. Each time the reader encounters a specific word, his or her mental image of it is strengthened. We say that the reader's 'lexicon' includes the mental image of that word, or, more precisely, that it includes the 'orthographic identity' of the word. The series of mental images of different words in one's lexicon is sometimes called the reader's 'sight vocabulary'. Having a capacious sight vocabulary is important for readers. It allows the reader to recognize a lot words on sight, without having to sound them out. Being able to recognize a lot of, or even better *most* of, the words in a given text gives the reader a high degree of 'automaticity' in reading. This automaticity is the hallmark of the skilled reader. Freed from the task of having to figure out which words are on the page before him, the skilled reader can devote his mental resources to comprehending what they mean (Wimmer, Mayringer og Landerl, 1998).

Comprehension refers to those higher cognitive processes that make it possible for the reader to extract the meaning of the text, to think about it, and to draw conclusions from it. These demanding tasks require that the reader has acquired the relevant real-life knowledge and experience. Unlike decoding, reading comprehension cannot be made automatic. It requires attention and cognitive resources in order to happen.

Decoding and comprehension are different types of skills, but in normal, skilled reading they work closely together. Research has conclusively shown that accurate and automatic word decoding is a necessary prerequisite for good reading ability (Adams, 1990). A deficit in word decoding will therefore hinder the reader's comprehension of the text. On the other hand, good comprehension skills will lend support to the decoding process, especially for young readers. Decoding and comprehension are therefore the two main subprocesses that good reading ability builds on, and both are necessary. Gough and Tunmer (1986) have expressed this in their 'Simple view of reading': *Reading = decoding x comprehension* Reading ability is the *product* of decoding and comprehension. If one of the factors is zero, then the product is zero. Good reading ability needs both.

In this book we will primarily be looking at the word decoding process. As mentioned, research has shown that a general poor reading ability is often caused by difficulty in decoding words rapidly and accurately, and poor word decoding ability is one of the major symptoms of that form of reading difficulty which is termed 'dyslexia'.

The question then arises, why do these pupils have such a hard time learning to decode words? In order to answer this question, we need to look at the different strategies involved in decoding and at the normal development of reading ability. It is also important to know about the different perceptual and linguistic processes taking place concurrently with the different decoding strategies, and which factors can hinder them (Siegel, 1993).

Decoding Strategies

There are several different strategies readers use to decode words, depending on whether the word appears in isolation or in context. If the word is seen alone, there are two main strategies to choose from: *The orthographic strategy* (which produces what we call *orthographic reading*) and *the phonological strategy* (yielding *phonological reading*). If the word appears in a context, then the reader can use various cues provided by the context. Nonetheless, the orthographic and phonological strategies are more important for good reading than contextual cues (Share and Stanovich, 1995).

The orthographic strategy allows the reader to decode the word immediately, that is, to go directly from the word's orthographic representation (the letter-sequence on the page) to the word's sound and meaning. In order to do this, the reader has to have seen the word a number of times before, so that he or she has established an orthographic identity for the word in the long-term memory. By 'orthographic identity' we mean *an inner, abstract representation of the word's spelling*. This is not an image of 'what the word looks like', because what words look like depends on a lot of extraneous things such as type face, style of handwriting, and so on. Instead, it is an abstract image or notion of how the word is spelled. In order to use the orthographic strategy, then, the reader has to have first acquired firm knowledge about the letters of the alphabet and how the alphabetic principle works.

In the literature this orthographic strategy is often called 'the direct route strategy' (Coltheart, Patterson and Marshall, 1980). When we read orthographically, all of the letters and their relative positions are crucial, but the letters are often mentally organized in higher-order structures, like word-stems, prefixes and suffixes, and common sequences of letters (Ehri 1991). For example, when reading the word *unexplainable*, the experienced reader probably 'sees' all of the letters both individually and in clumps: *un + explain + able*.

The orthographic strategy is what skilled readers generally use, because most of the words skilled readers encounter are words they have seen in print hundreds or thousands of times before. That is why they recognize them. But when the reader is confronted with an unfamiliar word, or an experimentally devised nonword, then he or she needs to use the phonological strategy (Share and Stanovich, 1995). When we read phonologically, we decode the word by breaking it down into letters or short segments of letters. These letter segments are first recoded into sound individually and then the sounds are blended together to create a smooth string of sounds. This string of sounds is the raw material used for recognizing the word.

In addition to the orthographic and phonological strategies, two fundamental ways of getting at the phonological identities of single words, there is a third strategy, the so-called *analogy strategy* (Glushko, 1979; Goswami, 1994). Here is an example: Let us say that a young reader has learned to recognize the word *hand*. This bit of knowledge can make it easier for him or her to decode the word *sand*. Seeing that the two words share the same last three letters, and being able to mentally substitute the *h*-sound with the *s*-sound, makes the decoding process easier. Here the pupil has used part of the phonological strategy (switching the *h* for the *s*), and the orthographic strategy (when recognizing the -*and* part of the word).

The strategies we have been looking at can be used when decoding both single words in isolation and words appearing in context. But the decoding of words that are presented in a context can also be made easier by the *semantic, syntactic* and *pragmatic cues* found in the context.

The *semantic cues* are the clues found in the content of the text. The word *doctor* is easier to decode when it appears in a sentence like: *The man got sick and had to go to the doctor.* We have reason to believe, however, that pupils who have acquired good decoding skills only to *a small degree* make use of the semantic cues when they decode words (Share and Stanovich, 1995). In fact, having to use the semantic cues of a text is a characteristic trait of poor readers. It appears that they use this strategy to compensate for their deficient orthographic and/or phonological abilities.

The *syntactic cues* make it possible for the reader to make an educated guess as to which class of word (noun, verb, conjunction, etc.) to expect in a particular position in the sentence, and how it probably is conjugated. For example, in the sentence: *I hope you can come,* the first four words create the expectation that the fifth word will be *come* and not *came*. These cues give some support to the decoding, but as with the semantic cues, readers who have solid decoding skills do not seem to use the syntactic cues very much.

The *pragmatic cues* are the hints and clues found things that 'surround' the text, such as pictures, the directions the teacher gave, the general situation, etc. These cues, like the semantic and syntactic cues, are thought to have some influence on the decoding process, but primarily they are important to the reader's comprehension.

Strategies that build on contextual cues are called *contextual strategies*, as opposed to *context-free strategies*.

How do the different word decoding strategies develop as the child learns to read? It seems that the child's reading development progresses in stages, and that the process typically begins before the child 'officially' starts learning to read at school. And as we shall see, the stages of reading development correspond to the decoding strategies we have described.

Stages of Reading Development

Right from the start we need to be clear about what we mean by 'stages' in children's reading 'development'. Reading is not a naturally occurring part of any child's development. Rather, it is a culturally determined activity, and as such it is influenced by teaching methods and the child's personal experiences with printed matter (Seymour and Evans, 1992). This means that what we call 'stages in reading development' are not claimed to be a set of firm, immutable stages all children go through, as is often the case with other 'stage theories' found in developmental psychology. In particular, we know that some children spend more time at a particular stage than others, and that a particular stage can be more important for one child than for another. Some children seem to jump over a particular stage, and we often find children at a mixed stage of development, where they mainly use the technique typical of one stage, but also rely on the techniques of an earlier stage in special circumstances.

In the literature we find several theories as to how reading ability develops through time (Chall, 1983; Ehri, 1992; Frith, 1985; Gough and Hillinger, 1980; Spear-Swerling and Sternberg, 1994). Our version of a model of the stages of reading development is presented in Figure 2.1.

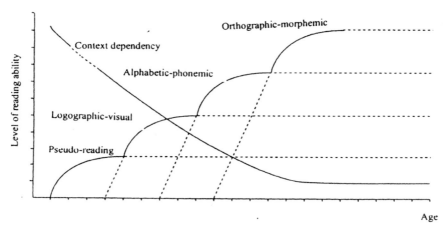

Figure 2.1. Stages in the development of word decoding. As children develop, their dependency on contextual cues diminishes. Broken lines indicate that a strategy is still available, even though it is not the preferred decoding strategy.

When children begin to learn to read, they are very dependent on contextual cues. This dependency diminishes throughout the child's development, as indicated by the line running from upper-left to lower-right.

As we see in the model, the development of the various strategies is not linear. The learning curve is steepest at the beginning of each stage, when the child catches on to the new technique rather quickly, and gradually flattens out as the skill is mastered. We assume that the child's skill remains intact, even though the skill is superseded by the next, more advanced technique. This way of looking at the development of children's decoding skills is in agreement with recent research (Francis et al., 1996).

Another aspect worth noting is that the types of reading overlap in time. When a decoding strategy has been successfully learned, it is not forgotten when the child acquires a more effective strategy; it persists as a back-up strategy that can be used when needed. The hallmark of the skilled reader is a flexibility in choice of decoding strategy. Even though the good reader recognizes most words immediately (what we call orthographic reading), there will always be some words he or she is encountering for the first time. Having a repertoire of other techniques at hand is no small advantage.

We suggest the following four stages in reading development:

1. Pseudo-reading
2. Logographic-visual
3. Alphabetic-phonemic
4. Orthographic-morphemic

Pseudo-reading

Young pre-schoolers usually have vague and sometimes confused notions about what writing is, and they tend to approach writing the same way they deal with other things and events. Occasionally it looks like a child is reading when he or she is really 'reading' the environment, not the writing itself. A good example of pseudo-reading was found in our study among Swedish-speaking preschoolers in Finland. Because of Finland's bilingual situation, many consumer products are printed with a Swedish-language label on one side, and a Finnish label on the other. As part of an interview, we showed them a common milk carton with the Swedish word for milk, *MJÖLK*, written in big letters on the side facing them. We asked the children what was written there, and all of them answered without hesitation *mjölk*. Then we surreptitiously turned the carton around so that the Finnish-language side with the word *MAITOA* facing front. When we asked them again what was written on the carton, most of the children answered: 'But I already told you. That says *mjölk*.' Even when we put two cartons beside each other, one with the Finnish side and the other with the Swedish side facing out, we found out that only those children who knew the names of many of the letters of the alphabet were able to determine that the cartons in fact had different words on the sides facing out.

Similar results have been reported by Masonheimer, Drum and Ehri (1984). In their study they systematically eliminated clues from the context. As long as the characteristic logo was present, for example McDonald's golden arches, the oval around the word *PEPSI*, Lego's characteristic type face, etc., the children were able to identify a lot of the words. But when the company name was presented in a normal type face, the scores sank dramatically. When the letters in a logo were tampered with, for example when they presented the Pepsi logo but respelled it *XEPSI*, only the children who knew the letters of the alphabet discovered the change. So it seems that children at this stage of reading development do not really look at letters *as letters*. Sometimes they do not seem to be aware of letters at all, but use the contextual clues and 'read' the environment.

Perhaps we should be asking why they should bother to look at the letters at all, when the context provides enough information for them to meet their needs. If they want a soft drink or a hamburger, why worry about spelling? How many of us adults can describe the details of, for example, the dials of our wristwatches, even though we look at them dozens of times a day? And what do we really know about the coins we use every day? Which of the famous people are on which of the coins or bank notes? The reason for our lack of awareness is simple: there is no reason for us to latch on to irrelevant details. We look at our watches to find out what time it is, and we look at our small change in order to pay for things. We should not expect children to attend spontaneously to details that are irrelevant for the purpose at hand. Awareness about and insight into the details of written language are things that have to be consciously taught by teachers or parents, because they know that these details will be of importance to the children as they mature and take their place in a literate society.

Children in our culture live in a world of print, a world where adults garner instructions and information from written matter every day, and where writing is highly valued. Nearly every child notices this. Most children in our part of the world are subjected to quite a bit of informal written-language socialization. Some parents systematically and energetically help their children discover writing (cf. e.g. Söderbergh, 1971), while others are less pushy. But nearly all children are in one way or another encouraged and coaxed to begin to be aware of writing as writing. The first word they learn to write is often their own name. Then they typically learn to recognize *MOM* and *DAD* and perhaps the name of a sibling or friend. They look at signs and labels. After a while, some children - long before they start their formal schooling - have learned to recognize an impressive repertoire of written words.

The logographic-visual stage

Most of our children are given some informal instruction in reading by parents, older siblings and friends prior to starting school. Thus, many preschoolers have learned to notice that the graphical details of a written word are what make it one word and not some other.

At the logographic stage children have not yet grasped the alphabetical principle, or as we often say, they have not yet 'cracked the code'. They treat each word as an independent stimulus, and learning to identify words is a kind of stimulus-response learning, a learning based on fairly simple associations between a graphical pattern (logographs) and the name of the word. The basic principle of alphabetic writing - the fact that a word's spelling is a representation of its sound - is secondary for the child, who pronounces the name of the word as soon at it is recognized. The order of the letters in the middle of the word do not normally affect the child's ability to recognize (correctly or incorrectly) the word. The word *CAMEL*, for example, may be recognized on the basis of the letter M, which may remind the child at this stage of a camel's two humps. Sometimes the length of a word will provide the child with a hint as to the word's identity, but the general contour of a word does not seem to provide the child with much usable information. In a study of children at the logographic stage, Seymour and Elder (1992) presented a number of words written in a jagged type face, or with the letters arranged vertically. The children were still able to recognize the words if they had previously learned them in their normal appearance.

The logographic reading strategy can best be characterized as learning to associate the visual traits of a word with its name. By using this strategy, the child is able to recognize many words even though he or she has not yet learned any letters. But as time goes by and the child needs to learn more and more words, this strategy proves unsuccessful. Latching on to unique visual traits for new words becomes more and more difficult, and the process breaks down. The child's logographic reading becomes increasingly marked by errors and wrong guesses.

Before children have learned to crack the alphabetic code, their logographic reading can be assisted by their knowing the names of the letters of the alphabet. Even though the names of the letters do not provide exact information as to the sounds the letters make, they nonetheless provide the child with valuable clues as to the sounds of a word. In a series of experiments, Ehri and Wilce (1985) have shown that knowledge of the letters makes word recognition easier long before the child has learned the alphabetical code.

Why can't children simply stay at the logographic stage and increase their reading vocabulary to an acceptable level? Learning to recognize words logographically would involve treating written words almost like Chinese ideograms. This obviously works for Chinese, but our alphabetical writing system is simply not designed for learning in this way. After a while, the risk of mixing up visually similar words becomes too great, and the whole effort is threatened with collapse. The whole point of our alphabetic system is that with 26 letters (give or take the few extra letters and diacritical markings found in foreign languages) we are able to represent the infinite number of utterances possible in spoken language. Treating each word as a unique graphic unit would be an unnecessarily cumbersome way of doing it. For example, decoding the words *write, wrote, written,* and *writing* and *writer* without utilizing the information provided in their spellings, would be a very uneconomical way of decoding.

Seymour and Evans (1992) grant logographic reading a more important function than is common among researchers. They claim that in time the logographic strategy develops into something more than mere stimulus-response association learning. As the child acquires knowledge about the letters, they think that this may provide the child with important cues that he or she can use in conjunction with the logographic strategy. More importantly, Seymour and Evans claim that the logographic strategy can serve as an adequate foundation for the development of *orthographic* reading, that is, some children may be able to develop good reading skills *without* really learning how to phonologically decode words (see

Seymour, 1990). This deviates from the traditional notion of sequence of stages in reading development, in which learning orthographic reading presupposes the ability to read phonologically (Frith, 1985). If Seymour and Evans are right, then this should change the way we teach remedial reading. Among other things, we will have to ask whether it is wise to spend time teaching the phonological strategy to pupils who show great difficulty in grasping it. Perhaps these pupils can be better taught by training them to associate the word's structure (its letter-sequence seen as a whole) with its pronunciation, instead of insisting that they 'sound it out' slowly, then blend the individual sounds into the word. But how can they develop a skill without exploiting the basic principle on which the skill rests?

The alphabetic-phonemic stage

The transition from the logographic to the alphabetic principle is a radical change in how pupils deal with written words. It flows from a completely new insight into what written words are, and it leads to a new attitude toward reading. Suddenly children need to look at words analytically, and they need knowledge about the connection between the shape of the letters (graphemes) and its sounds (phonemes). The hallmark of the alphabetic-phonemic stage is that the reader has broken the alphabetic code.

Frith (1985) claims that the child's early, spontaneous attempts at spelling are important to making the transition to this stage. These early spellings, even though they are unconventional and primitive, involve pulling the spoken word apart and producing an ordered sequence of letters that are meant to represent the word's sequence of sounds. When children do this, they show that they have grasped the idea that words are made up of letters in a certain order; that they are not logographs with a certain 'look'. Moreover, being able to isolate and attend to individual phonological segments and to manipulate letters is an important stage on the road to breaking the code, because it helps the child to gain access to the abstract phonemes. This needs some explanation:

In order to identify the grapheme-phoneme correspondence rules - that is, how a letter-sequence represents a sound-sequence - it is first necessary to be able to pick out the units of sound (phonemes) in a word as it are pronounced and the units of spelling (graphemes) in the word as it is written. Here we need to be clear about what phonemes and graphemes are, and are not. The phonemes of a language are not merely its sounds, but rather a higher-order, abstract representation of the sounds; not the sounds themselves, but rather their place in the sound system, as it were. Most languages have only a few dozen phonemes, but a nearly infinite number of sounds. Speakers and listeners make and hear probably tens of thousands of phonologically different sounds. But all of these tens of thousands of sounds are perceived as being instances of the few dozen phonemes. Here is an example. Both *cake* and *cookie* begin with the phoneme /k/. (In this book we follow the convention of presenting phonemes between slashes.) But if you listen carefully to the /k/ in these words, you discover that they sound quite different. The quality of the /k/ is colored by the vowel coming after it. In fact, if you analyze the two /k/-sounds with a modern oscilloscope, you find that they give radically different readings.

Nonetheless, in speech they are perceived as instances of the same phoneme. This is the miracle that makes language work, and it is the heart of the alphabetic principle. We return to this subject in Chapters 3 and 4, in connection with spelling and phonology.

Similarly, graphemes are not 'really' the letters used to spell words, but (in some sense) the abstract categories the letters belong to. It is a subtle distinction that goes like this: The letter *n* is an example of the grapheme *n*. The grapheme *n* is the category; it is the '*n*-ness' of all the particular instances of *n*'s, just as the /k/ is the '/k/-ness' of all the particular pronunciations of *k*. But the distinction between letters and the abstract graphemes they belong to is considerably less important than the distinction between phonemes and sounds, and we do no great conceptual harm in using the terms graphemes and letters interchangeably.

Generally speaking, graphemes code phonemes one to one. But often it takes more than one grapheme to code a phoneme. Examples would be the two graphemes *ph*, which usually encode the one phoneme /f/, and the four graphemes in the ubiquitous letter sequence *-ough*, which can encode either a single vowel-phoneme (as in *though*) or a vowel+consonant phoneme-sequence (as in *enough*). There is even an example of a grapheme that usually encodes *two* phonemes: the grapheme *x* is usually pronounced (in English as in many other languages) as /ks/.

In recent years the notion of *phonemic awareness* as been the focus of much research (e.g. Høien et al., 1995; Lundberg, Frost and Petersen, 1988; Torgesen et al., 1992). Phonemic awareness refers to the ability to mentally divide up a spoken word into its constituent phonemes: being able to hear, say, the word *hit* as /h/ + /i/ + /t/. There is ample empirical research from around the world that shows that there is a strong connection between phonemic awareness and reading ability (for an overview, see Share and Stanovich, 1995), and that phonemic awareness makes it easier for the child to grasp the alphabetic principle. This is a major theme in Chapter 4.

Some researchers claim that phonemic awareness is necessary in order for the child to achieve good phonological reading ability (Byrne and Fielding-Barnsley, 1993), while others claim that phonemic awareness is a *result* of having learned to read (Morais, 1991). Some claim that dyslexics have a poorer awareness of phonemes because they cannot read well, and therefore do not read much; while others claim than that dyslexics cannot learn to read because they lack phonemic awareness.

Perhaps we can get closer to the truth by looking at the development of phonemic awareness and reading development as two interactive processes: being good at manipulating phonemes makes it easier to learn to read, and being able to read leads to a strengthening of the pupil's phonemic awareness (Bradley and Bryant, 1985).

Even though the alphabetic-phonemic stage is the core of the reading development process, we lack firm knowledge as to exactly *how* the child breaks the code and learns to use the principle in a productive way. And when the child has managed to break the alphabetic code, there is still a long way to go until his or her decoding ability is fully developed. The beauty of this strategy is that it allows readers to pronounce words they haven't seen before. But this skill comes at a high cost: the alphabetic-phonemic strategy makes great demands on the reader's attention, leaving him or her less mental capacity to devote to understanding the text. Furthermore, when the decoding proceeds too slowly for a reader's working memory - which often happens when we laboriously sound out long words - the first sounds of a word are forgotten, or the first words in the sentence are forgotten, and the sentence is not comprehended. But because the alphabetic-phonemic strategy allows the reader to read new words, Jorm and Share (1983) call it 'a self-teaching model of early reading acquisition'. When using this strategy, the reader's attention is necessarily focused on the structure of the word, so the reader gradually learns how the word is spelled, which in turn makes it easier to decode it next time. Eventually the young reader will be able to recognize the string of letters correctly, effortlessly and without hesitation. This is the hallmark of the next and highest level of word decoding: The orthographic-morphemic stage.

The orthographic-morphemic stage

Gradually the child starts to discover patterns in the words he or she is learning. Where the child previously saw only a long string of letters that had to be sounded out one by one, the child now sees that many of the letters come 'prepackaged' in familiar chunks. For example, a child who encounters the word *treefrog* for the first time may well recognize the two parts, *tree* and *frog*, and thereby quickly reach the phonological identity of the word. Or, when encountering the word *bewitched*, the child may fairly quickly see the prefix *be-* (familiar in words like *because*), then see the word-stem *witch*, followed by the familiar past tense suffix *-ed*. The intimidating nine-letter word becomes a reader-friendly three-chunk word.

In cases like these, the child is utilizing the *morphemes* of language. Morphemes are word-stems, prefixes and suffixes, the smallest units of language that carry meaning. They are orthographic structures at a somewhat higher level of abstraction than the phonemes. This new way of decoding allows the decoding process to become fully automatic, fast and accurate, without the reader consciously having to sound out the phonemes of the word.

This type of reading is sometimes called 'whole-word reading,' but this term is misleading, a relic of a misunderstanding that was once prevalent among reading researchers. Orthographic-morphemic reading happens very fast: with only one fixation of the eyes we can take in 12 to 15 letters, and a fixation usually only takes about one-quarter of a second. These facts led many researchers to believe that good readers at this stage read words as whole units, without any mental work being done on the word's sequence of letters. A more modern view points out that the mind is capable of working very rapidly with sequences of letters, perceiving all of them, in the right order. It is just that they tend to fall into familiar chunks. Probably the only type of true whole-word reading done is the logographic-visual type of reading we discussed above. When we see the Coca-cola logo or the McDonald's sign, we recognize the sound-identity of the brand name instantly. If someone had changed one of the letters, but maintained the overall look of the logo, even a very skilled reader might not notice.

An automatic word decoding at the orthographic stage frees the reader's cognitive resources so that he or she can deal with the semantic and syntactical structures that make the text meaningful. This ultimately allows reading to become a kind of externally steered thinking.

We have now reached the highest level of word decoding ability, but readers at this stage still have a long way to go before they have acquired a fully developed reading ability. Really good, experienced readers are able to perform advanced interpretations, to draw conclusions and inferences from the text, to read different types of material in different ways, etc. These abilities draw upon yet higher mental processes which are, at this time, poorly understood (see Spear-Swerling and Sternberg, 1994).

Context and Word Recognition

In the development of word decoding and recognition, the young reader's dependence on contextual cues diminishes as the process becomes increasingly automatic (Fawcett and Nicolson, 1993; Yap and van der Leij, 1994a, b). At the early pseudo-reading stage the unique string of letters that makes up the word plays an insignificant role at most. Children at this stage 'read' the environment (context), not the words; for them, the context *is* the message. At the logographic-visual stage, children experience written words as visual patterns. But because they are only able keep a limited number of them sorted out in memory, their reading is marked by a lot of context-dependent guesswork: Perhaps the child decodes the initial letter of the unfamiliar word, then ventures a guess based on contextual clues in the text or in the illustration on the page.

Contextual cues can also help the child's decoding at the alphabetic stage. Seeing a picture of a dinosaur, and patiently sounding out *d-i-n-o-*, the clever reader will make the connection without bothering to sound out the remaining letters.

By when the reader has reached the orthographic-morpheme stage, context is not important and is rarely used. These readers have no problem attending to the -*s-a-u-r*. It costs them little time or energy. It happens faster than moving their eyes over to the illustration, then back to the text.

This view of the developing reader's diminishing reliance on context is richly supported by the data. But it is sharply at variance to the well-known and once-popular 'top-down' theories of Goodman (1976) and Smith (1973). According to proponents of the 'top-down' school, good readers use the context actively; in fact, truly excellent readers can extract so much information from the context that they need little in the way of input from the letter-strings on the page. For these readers, a glance at, say, the first letter or two of the word, and a glimpse of the word's general length and shape, combined with their expectations of what the word logically must be, is enough. They get the word right almost without seeing it. For 'top-down' proponents, reading, in a famous phrase, is a 'psycholinguistic guessing-game'.

It was an interesting theory, but there never was much in the way of data to support it. One possible reason for the promulgation of 'top-down' theories was a confusion between decoding and comprehension. Good readers, as we know, do make rich use of contextual information when they grapple with a text. But they use this information to comprehend the text, not to decode the words. What happens, it seems, is that the context, combined with their background knowledge of the subject, leads them to develop an hypothesis about the meaning of the text. This hypothesis is then corrected and refined by the meaning of the words they decode. In other words, good readers read actively. They fold the emerging text into their hypothesis, always trying, as we say in a particularly apt phrase, to 'make sense' of the text. But the skilled reader's word decoding process per se does not derive much support from the context.

We have been looking at some of the more important aspects of the basic word decoding strategies and the stages of reading development from the preschooler's early pseudo-reading to the automatic decoding that is the hallmark of the fluent, comprehending reader. We will take a closer look at the perceptual and linguistic processes which take place during decoding, but first we will attempt to visualize the decoding process in a model.

A Model of Word Decoding

Our word decoding model, shown in Figure 2.2, builds on the dual-route theory (Morton, 1979), which states that there are two paths or routes to the mental lexicon.

This model is a *word processing* model, that is, a model which shows the psychological processes taking place during the decoding of words in isolation. We could also say that it is a description of how a limited module for word decoding could be thought of as operating.

It is not a model of *all* the mental processes taking place when we read. Most importantly, the syntactical and most of the semantic aspects of the reading process are not shown, for two reasons. The first is that we do not yet know enough about how the reader's work with grammar and meaning is psychologically structured. We know some of the details of the story, but we have no sound theory as to how these enterprises are cognitively organized. Secondly, including grammar and meaning in the same model with word processing would make the diagram unwieldy. Our purpose in constructing the model and presenting it in a schematic diagram is to provide an overview.

The *orthographic strategy* is shown in bold-faced arrows, while the *phonological strategy* is shown in lighter ones.

The square in the middle symbolizes the *lexicon*. The lexicon is the location of our long-term memory for words. This is where we store our knowledge about how words (and sub-word units like prefixes and suffixes) are *pronounced*, what they *mean*, and how they are *spelled*. Processes here are memory processes.

The circles indicate the various psychological processes that take place when we use the orthographic or the phonological strategy. The arrows between the circles show how a bundle of information is relayed from one process to the next. The broken feedback lines from the lexicon to the individual processes show that the word processing at every point is also influenced by the reader's lexical knowledge. We have reason for believing that there are two-way connections between the individual processes, and this is shown in the model by the broken arrows.

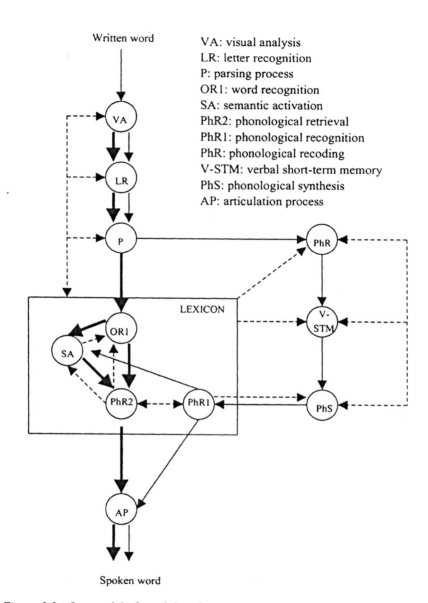

Figure 2.2. Our model of word decoding.
The orthographic strategy is indicated by the bold-faced arrows and the
phonological strategy by the lighter ones. The broken lines indicate feedback from
the lexical processes and the interaction between the separate processes.

The first three decoding processes, the Visual Analysis (VA), Letter Recognition (LR), and Parsing Process (P) are a part of both of the strategies, as are the Semantic Activation (SA) in the lexicon and the Articulation Process (AP) at the bottom of the model. A deficit in one of these processes will have a negative effect on both the phonological and the orthographic strategies.

Orthographic Word Recognition (OWR1) and Phonological Word Retrieval (PhWR2) are critical processes for the *orthographic strategy* only. A deficit in one of these will impair the reader's ability to recognize words 'on sight', but will not interfere with his ability to sound words out.

Four other processes are critical to the *phonological strategy* only, namely the prelexical Phonological Recoding (PhR), the verbal Short-Term Memory (STM), Phonological Synthesis (PhS), and the Phonological Word Recognition (PhWR1). A deficit in one or more of these four processes will have a negative effect on using the phonological strategy, but will not hinder using the orthographic strategy.

Let us now take a look at how the decoding process is thought to function. A word of warning, though. Word processing is a complex skill, and there are a lot of processes taking place. This means a model of the whole process will include a considerable number of arrows. So bear with us in this description, and make frequent reference to the diagram. This initial explanation will be brief. In subsequent sections we return to the many processes and flesh out the explanation.

When the reader looks at the written word, the first thing that happens is that he performs a Visual Analysis and Letter Recognition. These are *perceptual processes*, as opposed to all the subsequent processes, which are *linguistic processes*. Later in this chapter we will be taking a closer look at these two perceptual processes and what can go wrong with them, but for now it is enough to note that the output of the perceptual processes is information about the visual form of the word and the letters that constitute it.

This information is outputted to the Parsing Process (P). This is where the reader parses, or divides, the word into more manageable chunks, seeing e.g. the nine-letter *bewitched* as a three-morpheme word, for example.

The information about the word garnered from the Parsing Process is outputted in two directions: to the phonological strategy to the right in the diagram, and straight down to the orthographic strategy. We will first follow the orthographic route.

The information garnered from the Parsing Process is used by the Orthographic Word Recognition process (OWR1), where, optimally, the word is successfully recognized.

A point of contention here is whether it is necessary for the reader to identify all the letters in a word in order to recognize it. Our feeling is that if the word is very familiar to the reader, and if the reader has good reason for expecting that word to appear in this context, then information about the word's length, visual shape, and first few letters *can* be enough to trigger recognition. But normally, readers do take into account all the word's letters, even though the recognition process is very rapid. Recent research indicates quite conclusively that efficient and rapid word recognition is built on firm and automatic knowledge about all the letters in the word (Adams, 1990).

When the word has been recognized, the reader's activated orthographic knowledge causes his or her semantic knowledge to be activated (SA). The reader 'remembers' what the word means.

This semantic knowledge about the word, together with the orthographic knowledge, is used to search the phonological long-term memory in the lexicon during the Phonological Word Retrieval process (PhWR2). This triggers the reader's knowledge as to how the word is pronounced. This phonological knowledge then becomes the input of the Articulation Process (AP). The word is pronounced.

This is what happens, according to our model of the normal reading process, when the reader knows the spelling of the word.

If the reader does not recognize the spelling, then the orthographic route will be fruitless. To get around this block, the word processing takes a different route, the *indirect route*, where the reader uses the *phonological strategy.*

Backing up to the Parsing Process, we see that the information about how the word hangs together is also outputted to the Phonological Recoding process (PhR) Here, if the OWR1 process of the orthographic route draws a blank, the letter sequence gets converted into internalized speech sounds - the mental image of the sounds of the word. The resultant phonological segments are then stored briefly in the verbal Short-Term Memory (STM). Then these short segments are tied together to form a mental image of the sound of the whole word in the Phonological Synthesis process (PhS).

These three processes, which together are what we mean by 'sounding out words', are called *prelexical* processes, and the underlying apparatus is called the *prelexical system.* They are prelexical because they work with letter sequences that, for the time being at least, have no lexical value for the reader: They are just letter-strings which code pronounceable phoneme-strings. For all the reader knows at this point, the letters on the page may be a bogus nonword, a typographical error, or a word the reader knows but hasn't seen enough times in print for the spelling to sink in.

The result of the Phonological Synthesis process at PhS is outputted in two directions, to the lexical Phonological Word Recognition (PhWR1) process in the lexicon, and at the same time directly to the Articulation Process (AP). When the output arrives at the lexicon, the sound-image of the word is either recognized as a word the reader knows, or it is not recognized. If the sound *is* recognized, then its meaning is semantically activated (SA). If it is not recognized, no meaning pops up in the Semantic Activation, but it can at least still be pronounced because it was outputted to the Articulation Process directly from the Phonological Synthesis process (PhS).

As we have described the reading process, it may seem to some people like an elementary wiring-diagram, with a sequential series of neatly demarcated processes. In truth, reading involves a more complex relationship between the various subskills. Some of this is indicated by the broken arrows, which show the feedback paths. For example: all of the lexical processes provide some limited feedback and support to the three first processes, the Visual Analysis, Letter Recognition and Parsing. By this we mean that as soon as the reader looks at the word, his knowledge of the sounds, shapes, and meanings of words comes into play.

It is easier to perceive words that you know and half-way expect in the context of the passage. Furthermore, we have described the orthographic and the phonological strategies as two separate routes. They are, but they can take place at the same time. Generally, we use the orthographic strategy when we read, because we have already learned how most of the words we read are spelled. We recognize them on sight and don't need to sound them out. But there is reason to believe that the phonological strategy is in operation in the background most of the time. (If it is a well-developed skill, it doesn't take up very much of the reader's mental energies.) For skilled readers, it functions as a back-up system that springs to the forefront of consciousness to correct the occasional misidentification, or when the truly unfamiliar word turns up.

An important characteristic of this kind of word decoding model is that it clearly demarcates a special step in the decoding process which grants access to the lexicon *before* the interpretative work with the text begins. In other words, it explains 'bottom-up' reading, which is generally how we read. While it may occasionally be the case that the reader's understanding of the text as a whole helps in the task of decoding some of the words, we feel that these cases are relatively rare. Normal reading, as we have described it in our model, is only possible when the reader is able to efficiently decode words without using the context.

In the next two sections we will be looking at the perceptual and linguistic processes involved in word recognition, and point out some of the factors that can negatively influence them.

Perceptual processes

The raw material for the two perceptual processes, the Visual Analysis (VA) and Letter Recognition Process (LR1), are derived from the sensory process of vision. Therefore, we need first to say something about how we see.

The sensory process

The sensory process of vision receives sensations from external stimuli and relays them to the sensory center of vision in the brain (mainly located in the occipital lobes).

The sensory process is automatic, and it receives two *parallel* sets of information, one from each of the eyes, in the course of one fixation. A fixation is the time during reading when the eyes are for practical purposes not moving. Each fixation lasts about a quarter of a second. A deficit in the sensory process will have a negative influence on word decoding, because all the subsequent processes (perceptual, linguistic and cognitive) have to build on the sensations gathered and relayed on by the sensory system.

In connection with the sensory process used in reading, we will be looking at *vision problems, eye motion, iconic persistence*, and some of the unusual characteristics of the *pathways of the optic nerves*. (For a fuller discussion, see Humphreys and Bruce, 1989; Willows, Kruk and Corcos, 1993.)

1. Vision problems

Vision problems that can lead to reading problems are problems with acuity, field of vision and binocular vision.

Acuity of vision is a complex function. It is a measurement of the ability to discriminate fine details in visual stimuli. Acuity is sharpest at the center of the field of vision, the *fovea*. The foveal field covers about two degrees around the point of fixation. Just outside of the fovea we find the *parafovea*, the area from two to about six degrees around the fixation point. The area outside the parafovea is called *the peripheral field of vision.* The farther away from the fovea an object is seen, the less clear it appears. This is because the receptors of light in the eyes, the cones and rods, are densely packed on the retina in the foveal area, and are less dense farther away. Some dyslexic problems have occasionally been attributed to poor acuity. For example, Geiger and Lettvin (1987) found that dyslexics had relatively greater problems in identifying visual stimuli presented in the foveal area than in the peripheral area. Their study showed that dyslexics could improve their reading by learning to utilize their peripheral vision. A study that we carried out among normal and dyslexic eighth-graders in Stavanger, Norway, did not find support for this conclusion (Bjaalid, Høien and Lundberg, 1993).

Reduced visual acuity can be caused by many different things, such as optical refraction errors, organic trauma, or inadequate stimulation. A study of any normal population will probably reveal cases of near-sightedness, long-sightedness and astigmatism, in addition to age-related long-sightedness. Studies show that near-sightedness and astigmatism are not more prevalent among dyslexic children than in control groups. In fact, near-sightedness seems to be somewhat more common among good readers, while *long-sightedness* is a bit more prevalent among dyslexic pupils (Harris and Sipay, 1985).

The *field of vision* is the area the eyes can receive sensory impressions from in the course of a fixation. Reading starts with a fixation, lasting about 250 milliseconds. In the course of this brief moment the receptors in the eyes receive the sensory impression of the letters that fall within the fixation field. This impression is extinguished by the next impression from the following fixation, usually about 10 to 12 letters to the right. The location of the fixations determine which of the letters fall within the central fields, that is the fovea and the parafovea. This part of the text is the stimulus that the sensory process gets to work with. Studies have shown that there is on average nearly one fixation per word when reading (Just and Carpenter, 1980). This means that the visual sensory process usually works with stimuli at the level of words when decoding.

Each of the eyes has a left and a right field. The left field of vision of each of the eyes transmits its information to the right half of the brain for further processing, and the right field of vision of each of the eyes sends its information to the left hemisphere. Studies of patients with brain damage show that either the right or the left half of the can be damaged without the other half being affected, depending on which side of the brain the trauma is located. This is evidenced in characteristic mistakes in decoding words, with a high frequency of reading errors either at the beginning of the word (or group of words) or at the end of it (Riddoch and Humphreys 1983).

Binocular vision is what we have when the sensory impression from the two eyes is put together to form one image without blurring or 'seeing double'. This is a very complicated process, and many different subprocesses have to be functioning in order for the image to be sharp and unified (Stein, 1993). Measuring the angle of convergence between the eyes when they are at rest provides some information about how well a person's binocular vision functions. Lie (1989) claims that it is reasonable to assume that conditions of excitement and unstable binocular vision can lead to fatigue during reading, and that this can in turn lead to the child's avoidance of reading. This, of course, hinders the child in acquiring automatic word decoding skills (Lie, 1989). A higher frequency of vision problems (in particular poor binocular vision and long-sightedness) among dyslexics than among normal readers is also reported (Stein, 1993; Stein and Fowler, 1985).

Stein and Fowler (1982) studied whether there was any differences between poor readers and normal readers with regard to eye dominance and the ability to coordinate eye movement (two aspects of binocular vision). In their studies they used the Dunlop test of eye dominance and coordination (Dunlop, 1972). In a study of 80 dyslexics they found that about two-thirds of the subjects had not developed a dominant eye, while only one pupil in the control group lacked dominance. They also showed that dyslexics without eye dominance can develop it in six months by covering one of the eyes when reading (Stein and Fowler, 1985). Moreover, they found that poor readers more often than normal readers had difficulty in coordinating their eye movements. Full correction of vision problems makes it easier for poor readers to learn to read. Stein (1993) claims that poor binocular vision can explain why dyslexics often report that the letters seem to 'swim' or 'dance', and that they 'see double' or reverse the order of letters. He therefore recommends that dyslexic pupils cover one eye when reading, but this is still a hotly debated recommendation (Bishop, 1989).

Research on the relationship between reading problems and vision defects has arrived at glaringly different results. Two Scandinavian studies, the 'Bergen Project' (Aasved, 1988) and the 'Kronobergs Project' (Lennerstrand and Ygge, 1995) failed to find any greater prevalence of binocular vision problems or other vision defects among dyslexics than among normal readers. They conclude therefore that dyslexics' problems are not vision problems. It would seem that a great deal of research remains before we can say we have an adequate understanding of the how visual processes impact on reading. (For overview, see Willows, Kruk and Corcos, 1993.)

2. Eye movements

Eye movements can be recorded by measuring the electrical activity in the muscles that control the motion of the eyes, or more directly by measuring the reflection of infrared light from the cornea.

When reading, our eyes move across the page in a series of jerks. These *saccadic movements*, as they are called, take the eyes from one fixation point to the next. During the fixation the eyes are at rest, and this is when the visual information is experienced. About 90 percent of the time during reading the eyes are fixated (Rayner, 1997). Each saccadic movement lasts about 30 milliseconds and covers about two degrees, eight or nine letters under normal conditions. But the length varies according to the difficulty of the reading material. The saccadic movements are ballistic; that is, when they have been started, their speed, direction and length cannot be changed. The saccadic movements suppress the transmission of information from the fixation just before, and during the saccade no information can be obtained.

If the eyes 'land' on the wrong spot in the text, or if the text at the fixation point is not understood, then the eyes can take corrective action, for example *regressions*. Regressions are saccadic movements from right to left. Normally 10 to 25 percent of our saccadic movements are regressions, but the number of regressions depends on the level of difficulty of the text.

Many studies have shown that dyslexics have poorer eye movements, marked by many unsystematic saccadic movements. Pavlidis (1991a, 1991b) found that dyslexics exhibited more frequent and less smooth regressions than did normal readers. The regressions of the dyslexics lasted longer and went farther back in the text, giving their movement pattern a characteristic 'backwards stepping' motion - the mirror image of the normal pattern. Pirozzolo and Rayner (1978) have also described a dyslexic who had a typical backwards stepping eye pattern, but this was eliminated when he read the text backwards, that is rotated 180 degrees. Regression patterns are also found in adult normal readers who try to read a very complicated text.

This raises the question of which is the cause, and which the effect. Unsystematic saccadic motions can be a symptom of poor reading ability, or they can be the cause. An overview is found in Olson and Forsberg (1993). They found no difference in movement pattern during reading when they compared pupils who read poorly with younger pupils at the same level of reading ability.

Studies have been made of eye motion under experimental conditions where there is no demand made on reading skill. Pavlidis (1981) and Martos and Vila (1990) used points of light that were lit up successively from left to right, and the subjects were asked to follow the lights with their eyes. They found that dyslexics had many more unsystematic movements than normal readers, which leads them to claim that dyslexia is associated with unsystematic eye movements. A common weakness of these two studies is the small number of subjects in the experimental and control groups. Other researchers have carried out equivalent studies with larger groups of dyslexics without finding a higher degree of unsystematic movements among dyslexics, when level of reading ability is controlled for (see Olson and Forsberg, 1993).

Today there is no doubt that dyslexics exhibit more aberrant eye motion than normal readers at the same age level. The pattern of eye motion of the dyslexics resembles that of the beginning reader: the fixations last longer, the saccadic movements are shorter and greater in number, and there are more regressions. But most researchers would claim that this deviant pattern is not the real cause of the pupils' dyslexia. It is more reasonable to think that the deviant pattern seen in dyslexics and beginning readers merely reflects the difficulty of the decoding task (Olson and Forsberg, 1993). There are people who have serious disturbances in their eye movements (congenital nystagmus), who nonetheless learn to read well. For more research on eye-movements during reading, see Pollatsek (1993) and Kennedy (1993).

3. Iconic persistence

The end result of the sensory process is a stimulation of the receptors and the primary sensoric center in the brain. The condition of being stimulated persists a short while after the stimulus itself is gone, and in vision this phantom-like condition is termed *iconic persistence* (Høien, 1979). This iconic persistence is the basis of a sensory memory system called *iconic memory*.

The iconic memory has a large capacity, but a short life (about one-quarter of a second). An image stored in the iconic memory is wiped out by the next impression. The duration of the iconic memory can vary somewhat from individual to individual, and this difference may affect the subsequent processing of the sensory stimulus (Breitmeyer, 1993; Høien, 1979).

Høien studied the duration of iconic memory in a group of poor readers and a control group of normal readers. Two flashes of light with a very short interval between them were presented to each of the subjects. They were asked whether they saw one flash or two. A significantly greater number of poor readers 'saw' only one flash. Several subsequent studies have arrived at similar results (Lovegrove et al, 1986). What could be happening is this: an iconic persistence that has a longer duration than normal could lead to poor reading if the iconic memory of one word is masking the perception of the next word.

Lovegrove and Williams (1993) found that poor readers scored better on reading tests when the contrast between letters and background was reduced, for example by putting a blue or gray sheet of plastic over the page. According to their theory, reducing the contrast reduces the masking effect. Recent findings indicate that the duration of the iconic memory can be a result of certain features of the pathways of the optic nerves, which transmit the information gathered by the eyes to the brain. We return to this in Chapter 6; here we will merely present some of the main features of these neural pathways.

4. Characteristics of the neural pathways to the brain

There are two parallel systems in operation during the transmission of sensory information from the eyes to the perceptual and cognitive processing in the brain. These systems are termed the parvocellular system (P) and the mangocellular system (M). The two systems have different tasks to perform. The P system is involved in our ability to perceive details and colors, and there are a lot of P neurons in the central part of the field of vision (the fovea). The M system, on the other hand, gathers its information from the entire field, and it is especially active when the sensory input is very brief. This is characteristic of what we see when we read: groups of letters 'flash' by, never lingering, in fluent reading at least, for more than the bat of an eye. The reader has to decode a given word in about a quarter of a second, before trailing his or her eyes on the next word.

Both systems are important to reading (Breitmeyer, 1993). The P system provides the detailed information, while the M system, which is activated during the saccadic movement, interrupts the activity in the P system, thereby hindering the masking of the next set of visual input. Recent research has shown that dyslexia may be associated with a deficit in the M system (Livingstone et al., 1991; Hogben, 1997). These researchers have also found abnormal cellular structures in the M system of the brains of deceased dyslexics.

Visual analysis (VA)

Several factors determine the results of the perceptual process. First of all, the visual quality of the thing being looked at determines how well you perceive it. A poorly illuminated page will be hard for anyone to read. Secondly, the length of the individual's iconic persistence determines in part how long a span of time his or her perceptual system is allowed to use in processing the information.

Taylor and Taylor (1983) claim that the perceptual process actually consists of two subprocesses that work with the information in very different ways: the *holistic process* and the *analytical process.*

The holistic process works on the form of the stimulus. It is fast: its work is done in 50 milliseconds. When we read, the holistic process is envisioned as gathering information about the characteristics of the length and shape of the word, and perhaps its first and last letter.

The analytic process, according to Taylor and Taylor, works more slowly, taking about 200 milliseconds to do its job. It gathers information about the letters in the word - which ones are present and in what order. This analytic process is important to our ability to discriminate between words that have roughly the same shape.

Both of these processes are thought to be important to the reader's ability to quickly and accurately perceive words. A deficit in one of them will hinder perception and evidence itself in characteristic types of reading errors, according to Taylor and Taylor. More particularly, both of the processes are necessary for the pupil to be able to use the direct route strategy. If Taylor and Taylor's theory is correct, then we can also expect that the balance between these two processes can be harmed through genetic conditions and/or environmental factors.

There are in particular four factors that can affect the balance between the holistic and the analytic processes:

1.   the reader's cognitive style
2.   emotional problems
3.   attention deficits
4.   teaching methods

The reader's *cognitive style* is his or her characteristic way of working with information. Some readers are impulsive and react before they have analyzed the

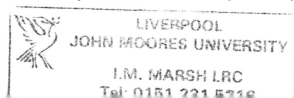

stimulus. They construct their perception by the fast holistic process and do not wait for the results of the slower analytic process. Other readers are more reflective. They do not answer until they have analyzed the stimulus. This reflective style does not dare bet on the speedy results from the holistic process, preferring instead to wait until the trusty analytic process has finished. This is how the reader's cognitive style may influence whether he or she constructs perceptions holistically or analytically, or both, depending on the type of text to be read and the reader's level of ability.

Emotional factors can also disturb the balance between the two processes. For some readers, emotional problems can limit the field of perception, thus hindering the use of the holistic process and forcing the reader to rely on brute analysis. This will evidence itself in difficulty in using the direct route strategy and in a greater dependence on the indirect route, creating readers who habitually and laboriously sound out the words.

Other readers with emotional problems will show the opposite tendency. They do not dare to take the necessary time to sound out the words analytically, and rely instead on quicker holistic processing. Their reading is marked by frequent errors and guesswork based mainly on the available semantic clues. We should note, however, that there are two different types of impulsiveness, one caused by the reader's emotional condition, and one that is the result of his or her cognitive style, previous learning experience, or both.

Attention deficits can also adversely affect the perceptual process. In the course of one fixation the reader has to attend to different parts of the field. An attention deficit can make it difficult to efficiently and systematically gather information from the whole field. It is possible that part of learning how to read consists of learning how to attend to texts in productive ways from moment to moment.

Closely related to the notion of attention is the concept of *filtering*. Readers need to attend to the letters when reading, but to do this productively they have to be able to filter out the inessential aspects of the letters, the better to concentrate on what really counts. Inessential aspects are such things as their color, peculiarities of the type face, the fly-speck on the page, etc.

Teaching also affects the balance between holistic and analytic reading strategies. Some pupils are taught not to make mistakes; precise decoding is considered an absolute necessity. Other pupils are encouraged to use contextual cues to make the decoding easier. For them, decoding is more than an analysis of the stimulus word.

These four factors - cognitive style, emotional condition, attention deficits and teaching methods - do not only affect the balance between holistic and analytic strategies in reading, but most likely in other types of tasks as well. They may influence the result of e.g. aural perception, as well as other types of problem-solving.

In the letter recognition process, to which we shall now turn, both the holistic and the analytic process play an important role.

Letter recognition process (LR)

Being able to accurately recognize written words requires a fast and automatic ability to recognize the letters that make up the word.

When pupils learn the letters of the alphabet, they learn about the unique set of characteristics that each of the letters has. Mixing up letters that have similar forms, for example *b* and *d*, may be due to difficulty in performing visual analysis, or it may simply be due to a lack of knowledge about which graphic feature defines which letter. Learning to discriminate successfully among letters can be achieved only through a conscious studying of them, and teachers need to devote a lot of classroom time to this subject. For example, the common *b-d* confusion is usually the result of a lack of knowledge about the importance of direction in letter identification.

Some pupils have special difficulties in learning the letters. Recent studies show that multi-sensory methods are especially valuable for these pupils (Hulme, 1987). We return to these methods in Chapter 8.

The process of recognizing letters is also supported by feedback from the letter's phonological identity. When a letter's written form (for example *S*) is associated with its name ('ess') and/or the sound it typically makes (/s/, /z/), then the perception of this letter will trigger these other identities, which in turn provides supportive feedback to the letter recognition process.

Similarly, if the child has learned to associate a letter with some semantic content - for example the letter *S* with 'snake' - then this association provides feedback to the letter recognition process. Associating *S* with a picture of a snake and the word *snake* is what we call visual-semantic-phonological support. Associating *S* with 'sun' is a purely sound-based association, which provides phonological-semantic support.

When several letters appear in the stimulus at the same time, identifying them can be done *sequentially* or *simultaneously*. When letters are identified sequentially, they are fixated upon one at a time; when they are identified simultaneously, the reader fixates on the whole group of letters at once and identifies them as a group.

Simultaneous letter recognition makes it possible for the reader to build up a network of associations between the letters. These are called *interletter associations* (see Adams, 1990). When the reader has seen a commonly occurring group of letters often enough, a separate orthographic identity for the group is established in the reader's memory. This in turn allows the reader to acquire firm knowledge about syllables, morphemes, and words.

Pupils who have difficulty with grapheme-phoneme associations (i.e. knowing which sounds particular letters usually represent) will also have problems with establishing good interletter associations. These pupils fixate on the individual letters so long that the letter's visual percept has disappeared before the next letter is perceived. Hence they do not see the 'forest' (the letter group) for the 'trees' (the individual letters). These pupils can often be best taught by getting them to focus on the highly frequent combinations of letters at the same time as they are being taught the individual letters.

Interletter associations also provide the good reader with feedback during the process of letter identification. When the reader perceives a syllable or a short word as a whole, then both the individual letters and the interletter associations are activated. Each of the letters also receives stimulation from the other letters in the group, and this is why single letters are easier to perceive in a well-known word than in isolation (Adams, 1990).

Normal word decoding is only possible for readers who are good at simultaneous letter identification. For good readers this is not an attention-demanding, analytical process in which the letters are identified and decoded one by one, but rather a swift, automatic process in which the syllable or word is perceived as a whole, and decoded in one full swoop. Readers who only perceive letters sequentially, and who therefore have no repertoire of interletter associations to draw upon, cannot do this.

Studies of patients with alexia, the reading problems which formerly good readers acquire after certain types of strokes and the like, give us reason to believe that the difference between holistic and analytic word decoding has a neurological basis. Some patients exhibit a loss of the ability to identify letters simultaneously. This is called *simultaneous alexia* (Legaard, 1987). These patients are unable to decode words orthographically, and have to rely on a laborious, letter by letter sounding out of even very familiar words. Their holistic processing is damaged, but their analytic processing is intact. The opposite pattern is found in patients with *attention alexia* (Shallice and Warrington, 1980). This form of alexia is characterized by the patient being able to read whole words, without being able to identify its letters. Their analytic processing is damaged, but their holistic process is intact.

Not only do letters have to be identified correctly, they have to be identified in the correct order. The words *from* and *form* are made up of the same letters; it is the order of the letters which determines which word is which. Some young readers make a lot of letter reversals. For them it is often found that improving the typography, e.g. making the letters larger or putting more space around them, can help them decode better. When working on texts without the more generous typography they need, these pupils seek to avoid making reversal errors by slowing down the pace of their letter recognition. This helps their decoding result, but devastates their comprehension.

Linguistic Processes

Parsing (P)

The process of *parsing*, or segmentation, as it also is called, is the process whereby words are mentally broken down into more manageable orthographic segments of various lengths - single letters, clusters of letters, syllables, or morphemes.

The parsing process uses the letters of a word as raw material, and brings to bear upon them the reader's acquired knowledge of the interletter associations - the experienced reader's 'feel' for which letter-clusters are highly frequent in the written language and which are less common or even impossible. The more frequently a certain letter combination has been associated with a certain pronunciation, then the stronger the association between the orthographic and the phonological segment becomes.

Here, too, diagraphs like *th* and *ph* are perceived as common, recognizable grapheme-pairs that code only one sound, and not two, as the very inexperienced reader might think. Moreover, the reader locates here the syllable-boundaries in long words. Good readers at the orthographic-morphemic level have the ability to see quickly where syllable-breaks are. For example, when the skilled reader sees the letter combination *-sr-* in the middle of a word, he or she knows intuitively that the *s* is at the end of one syllable and the *r* is the start of the next one. Why? Because that is how English spelling and phonology work. There are no English words with the phoneme-sequence /sr/ in the same syllable, and therefore there are no words with that spelling. When you see an word with the spelling *-sr-*, you can be sure that the letters are somewhere in the middle of a word with two (or more) syllables, like *classroom*. Either that, or the word in question isn't English, like the name of the country *Sri Lanka*.

Goldblum and Frost (1988) have shown that the parsing process is more sensitive to the structure of the syllables than to the word's morphology. Parsing happens automatically as the word is being perceived; it is not normally the result of a conscious decision on the part of the reader. Experience has shown that it is usually futile to give pupils a list of rules for how to segment words into syllables (Mewhort and Campbell, 1981). But it is useful, nonetheless, to focus the pupils' attention on the syllables of words, to train them to pick out syllables, and to emphasize syllable reading during the decoding of long words and nonwords. Skilled readers' ability to decode long words depends on their ability to segment words into syllables during the parsing process.

Recent research has also shown that knowing how syllables are constructed of 'onsets' and 'rimes' can help readers decode words (Treiman, 1992). Onsets are the initial consonant or consonant-cluster of a syllable; rimes are the syllable's vowel and any consonants that come after the vowel. For example, in the word *drags* the *dr-* is the onset, while *-ags* is the rime. A good way of teaching reading in the early grades is to present words in 'families' that share the same rime or onset. *Fat, bat, cat* can be taught together by pointing out that they have the same rime, just different onsets. We return to this method in Chapter 8.

Elbro (1990) has documented the critical role the reader's awareness of a word's morphemes plays in skilled word decoding, and he has shown that dyslexics often have a poor awareness of the morphemes of written language. Training pupils to recognize the most common morphemes should therefore be an important part of remedial programmes.

Word recognition process (OWRl)

When the reader has seen a word a number of times, an orthographic memory image or representation of the word is built up in the long-term memory in the lexicon. This image makes it possible for the reader to recognize the word when it is presented.

This construction of the visual memory image is mediated by the perceptual processes, which draw upon the distinctive features of the word. It is as if the mind constructs a list of distinctive features for each word that the reader learns to recognize, a list including all the unique characteristics which distinguish this, and only this, word. The construction of this list takes place through experiencing the word enough times, and the reader needs to encounter the word many times before the list for that word is complete. The list of distinctive features for any word includes such things as the general form and length of the word, and especially the unique set of letters and their order. Therefore, rock-solid knowledge of the letters is an absolute requirement for being able to acquire well-specified orthographic identities.

Skilled readers recognize words through a fast, automatic and parallel processing of the word's letters. In the orthographic memory in the lexicon, the word's letters are associated with each other, forming a tight orthographic unit. This allows the word to be recognized holistically, as a unit. The strength of the interletter associations is determined by the word's frequency in the language that the child has experienced in his or her reading 'career'. Highly frequent words have strong interletter associations that make them relatively easy to decode as a unit, while the opposite is true for the words of low frequency in the child's experience. They look and feel a bit odd, perhaps, and do not hang together well.

Semantic activation (SA)

Word recognition (OWR1) leads to semantic activation (SA), the process by which the reader understands the word. If the reader does not understand a word after it has been recognized orthographically, this can be due to three things: a lack of semantic knowledge, difficulty in activating semantic knowledge, or a rupture in the connection between the word's orthographic and semantic identities. These problems, however, are very rarely found when working with dyslexics. They are mainly seen in working with alexics (Coltheart et al., 1980).

There is reason for believing that the semantic processing starts before the orthographic processing of the whole word is finished. Semantic activation can take place with morphemes, because they have semantic identities; they 'mean' something. As soon as the parsing process has picked out a morpheme, it can be outputted to the semantic processor in the lexicon, which in turn can lend support to the rest of the orthographic processing of the word.

Phonological word retrieval (PhWR2)

The word's phonological identity can be activated either through the direct influence of the orthographic word recognition process (OWR1) or through semantic activation (SA). In normal reading either or both of these processes can be used for the phonological retrieval (PhWR2) of the word, but the direct connection between OWR1 and PhWR2 is probably the more important. At any rate, this route is the only possible route for words that have no semantic identity for the reader, words he or she has never seen nor heard, for example nonwords. On tests of word decoding we often find pupils who are much better at decoding content words (words with a good 'dictionary meanings' such as nouns, verbs, etc.) than they are at decoding function words (semantically 'empty' words like *the*, *an*, *of*). This discrepancy indicates that these readers have to use their semantic knowledge in order to retrieve a word's phonological identity.

Even though good readers do not have to phonologically recode words in order to access the word's semantic identity, the phonological recoding process nonetheless plays an important part in reading. First of all, phonological recoding allows single words to be stored in the working memory while the next words are being decoded. This is necessary in order to tie together groups of words into sequences that are meaningful. Secondly, the phonological recoding, perhaps especially of sub-word units like syllables and common letter-clusters, is an important back-up system for the word decoding process, especially for words of low frequency or words that are unknown to the reader (Adams, 1990). This phonological back-up mechanism can provide the processing system with a bit of additional information that helps it achieve a fast and accurate decoding.

The articulation process (AP)

Activation of the word's phonological identity leads to an activation of the word's articulatory identity. These two identities, the phonological and the articulatory, are so tightly connected that it is difficulty to imagine a situation where only one of them is activated. Because they are so closely connected, we would also expect that a well-established articulatory identity will help the corresponding phonological identity become established in the lexicon as the child learns to read, and that it helps activate the phonological identity when it needs to be recalled when reading.

Activation of the articulatory identity is a necessary prerequisite for the articulatory process. When a word is articulated, the 'set of directions' embedded in the word's articulatory identity is carried out. Difficulties in articulation can be traced back to a deficit in the set of directions itself, or to a deficit in the central or peripheral organs used in speech.

Prelexical phonological recoding (PhR)

This is the first step in the specifically phonological route; it is what the reader has to rely on when the letter-string is not recognized as a familiar word. The prelexical phonological recoding process (PhR) is a sequential process which turns the orthographic segments (letters and letter combinations) into phonological segments, mental sounds that correspond to the orthographic segments. This process has to work on the word in the right direction, from left to right. We term it 'prelexical' because it takes place before the process enters the lexical area.

In order for the Phonological Recoding process to be successful, the reader has to have acquired knowledge as to the phonological identities of the orthographic segments. The reader learns these by having the orthographic identities presented with their common phonological identities a number of times, so that strong associations between the two are established.

When reading, we recode the written text's graphemes into the spoken language's phonemes in accordance with the so-called grapheme-to-phoneme conversion rules. For a language such as English that is 'hard to spell' or is thought to be 'not very phonetic', these conversion rules are very complex, and sometimes even skilled readers will have to think twice about which conversion rule to apply. Some conversion rules are very simple. For example, a written word that starts with a *b-* is invariably pronounced with a word-initial /b/. But words *ending* in *-b* are a bit more difficult. Sometimes the *b* is pronounced (*tab, crib*) and sometimes it is silent (*climb, dumb, limb, succumb*). The reader has to choose which rule to apply. (Skilled readers will notice that the next-to-last letter is *m*; in the more complete set of conversion rules they use, they have the rule that states that words ending in *-mb* get pronounced /m/, so this is not a problem for them. Given the nonword *Semb*, they will read it off with a silent *b*.)

The prelexical system cannot readily perform a correct recoding of irregular words. By 'irregular words' we mean those words whose correct recodings use comparatively rare conversion rules, or whose recodings are unique. What often happens is that these words get converted in accordance with a more common rule, as if they were regular. In these cases, we say that the prelexical system regularizes the irregular words. A pupil who reads off the word *Thames* with a initial th-phoneme has regularized the pronunciation, that is, he or she has followed the more common conversion rule for *th-*.

The lexical system deals with all the words that are familiar to the reader; they do not have to been phonologically recoded (but may be anyway). The *prelexical system* can turn any acceptable letter sequence into internal speech sounds. By 'acceptable' we mean 'acceptable according to the *phonotactic rules.*' This needs some explanation:

In English there is no word spelled *wug*. But there could have been, because this letter sequence conforms to the English language's *orthotactic* rules for how words can be spelled. Moreover, the reader has no trouble pronouncing it, because the letter sequence points unambiguously to the *phonotactically acceptable* sequence of sounds *wuh-uh-guh*, which are effortlessly tied together to form *wug*. Again, there is no word that sounds like *wug* in English, but there could have been. So the prelexical system has no problem with forming a sound image for 'words' like *wug*.

On the other hand, a letter string such as *szokrlafj* does not look like a word in English, because it contradicts the orthotactic rules which state e.g. that acceptable words in English cannot begin with the letter sequence *sz-* nor end in *-fj*. More to the point, the letter string is phonotactically unacceptable because even if you patiently try to sound it out, you get a jumble of sounds that cannot be tied together in that order to form a phonotactically acceptable word in English. The sounds the letters ostensibly point to (according to the usual grapheme-to-phoneme conversion rules) contradict the phonotactic rules of English on several counts, so no sound image can be formed and the prelexical system gives up. Phonotactically and orthotactically acceptable 'words' like *wug* are called 'nonwords.' They are often used experimentally to test decoding ability precisely because they look like real words, but have zero semantic, phonological or orthographic identity. They can only be dealt with by the prelexical system.

As we see, the process of prelexical Phonological Recoding does many of the same things that the lexical coding processes in the lexical area, PhWR1 and 2, do. But the prelexical recoding is more labour-intensive. First of all, it has no semantic identity which can support it. Secondly, the phonological recoding makes great demands on the verbal Short-Term Memory (STM).

Verbal short-term memory (STM)

The capacity of the verbal short-term memory is critical for how many sound segments can be effectively handled by the synthesis process (PhS). We know that many dyslexics have poor short-term memories. This should be taken into account when their remedial programmes are devised, for example by teaching them to deal with orthographic elements larger than phonemes. This would give them fewer items to keep track of, even though each item consisted of more than one phoneme. We also know that factors such as emotional problems and attention difficulties can also truncate the short-term memory (cf. Lyon and Krasneger, 1996).

Phonological synthesis (PhS)

This is the process whereby the recoded phonological segments are bound together in a unified sound image that is similar enough to the pronunciation of the word for the reader to be able to access the word's sound identity in the lexicon. The synthesis process is thought to begin before the Phonological Recoding is finished. Nonetheless, the synthesis process depends on the Short-Term Memory, which stores the phonological segments after they have been recoded, while they are waiting to be drawn together to make a word.

Difficulties with the synthesis process can often be traced back to a poorly automated grapheme-phoneme recoding (PhR), a poor verbal Short-Term Memory, or to poor strategies in using the memory. But putting together a series of separate phonemes is not easy in itself. To see how hard it is, compare the pronunciation of the word *spill* with the phonemes /s/ + /p/ + /i/ + /l/. The phonological recoding of a word yields a jerky, very unwordlike phoneme sequence. Being able to make the sound of a real word out of a string of phonemes demands insight into how phonemes are co-articulated (Liberman, 1997). We return to the phenomenon of co-articulation in Chapter 3, in connection with spelling.

When the reader pulls the phonemes together successfully, this activates the word's phonological identity (PhWR1), which leads to the activation of the word's semantic identity (SA). The word is understood.

Objections to Dual-Route Models

The model presented in Figure 2.2 gives us a useful starting point for the mapping out of the various subprocesses involved in word decoding. One objection to this model is that it is based on the idea of two separate routes to the lexicon (Humphreys and Evett, 1985). It is therefore not able to account very well for the interaction between the orthographic and the phonological information at different levels, such as the level of single letters, syllables, morphemes, and words (Ehri, 1992).

In a recent article we have tried to address these objections (Bjaalid, Høien and Lundberg, 1997). It is important, however, to emphasize that any attempt at visualizing the complex psychological processes taking place during reading will, to greater or lesser degree, always present a simplified and therefore somewhat misleading picture of reality. We do not claim that the model presented in this chapter can provide us with satisfactory answers to all the complicated questions we may want to ask about word decoding, nor does it represent everything that we know about the process. We do, however, make the more modest claim that this model gives us a theoretical basis for further empirical studies, and that it functions well as a diagnostic tool. We return to the model's utility in diagnosis work in Chapter 7.

Connectionistic Theory - an Alternative to Dual-Route Models

In recent years researchers have begun to simulate the word recognition process on computers. They envision that decoding in the mind is carried out by the activity of a great number of processing units (neurons), and this process has been successfully modeled in computer programmes. In the programme, these units are grouped together in various fields or processors, e.g. phonological, orthographic, semantic and context-based processors. In addition the 'connectionist' researchers postulate a field for 'hidden units', which are responsible for providing feedback to the other fields. Each of the elements in this 'virtual brain' is connected to all the others through a network of *associations* or links, the quantitative value of which gets changed by the programme as it 'learns' to read. When the researchers 'teach' the computer programme to 'read' a given word, the programme quantitatively strengthens some of the associations, while others are allowed to languish. Each time the programme is presented with a word, the correct associations become stronger, and after a number of encounters with the word, the programme has 'learned' to recognize it.

After some training, the programme is able to recognize words in, to all outward appearances, the same way as human readers learn to read. Among other things, a given word's frequency and other linguistic factors will affect the programme's ability to learn to recognize it in very much the same way as these factors influence the human reader's recognition ability. In 'connectionistic' models like this, there is no lexicon, nor is there any separate 'route' for phonological recognition. Knowledge about words is represented only by the quantitative 'weights' on the connections between the processing units that code letters and phonemes.

Seidenberg and McClelland (1989) theorize that dyslexics have fewer 'hidden units' for word decoding than normal readers. Their theory is based on the fact that computer programmes with an experimentally reduced number of these hidden units show the same deficient ability to read words and to learn new words as do dyslexic pupils.

In the years to come we have good reason to expect that the efforts at computer modeling of reading will shed a lot of light on reading problems. But for the time being these connectionistic models have not been sufficiently studied for their results to have much practical import. Until such studies have been done, we will have to content ourselves with the kind of model shown in Figure 2.2, which has proved to be of help in diagnosing and remediating dyslexia.

Decoding Strategies used by Dyslexics

Because dyslexia is caused by a deficit in the phonological area, we would expect that dyslexics will have special difficulty in learning to use the phonological strategy, and that their phonological difficulties will also hinder them in acquiring well-specified orthographic identities. Because the teaching of beginning reading in our societies is often based on phonetic-based methods (phonics and the like), a deficit in the phonological area will soon show itself in the reader's inability to tie sounds together into words. The reading behavior of a particular dyslexic pupil will nonetheless vary somewhat from other pupils with similar problems, depending on which strategy he or she prefers using. Some poor readers stagnate at the 'sounding out' stage, even though this strategy leads to many reading errors. Others try to compensate by using alternative strategies.

It is not unusual to find dyslexics who use the logographic strategy, even though their classmates have moved on to far more fruitful ways of decoding. The logographic strategy allows them to recognize a certain number of words, and this can postpone the day when the teacher realizes that they can't really decode at all. The logographic strategy alone is never enough to make a good reader. But the question is whether it might form an adequate basis for learning the orthographic strategy, without having to go through the thorny prelexical Phonological Recoding process.

The developmental model shown in Figure 2.1 has been used to explain the various forms of dyslexia. Frith (1985) views dyslexia as a stagnation in reading development, and because different poor readers stagnate at different stages, we have different types or subgroups of dyslexics. A stagnation at the logographic-visual stage, according to Firth, leads to the reader becoming a 'phonological dyslexic'. Phonological dyslexia is characterized by a difficulty in tying sounds together into words. A stagnation at the alphabetic-phonemic stage leads to a reader becoming an 'orthographic dyslexic'. This type of dyslexia is characterized by a difficulty in learning how words are spelled, which in turn hinders the acquisition of rapid and accurate word recognition.

According to Frith, reading development proceeds according to immutable stages. Learning to decode at one stage presupposes that the reader has achieved good ability at the former stage. This understanding of reading development implicitly denies that pupils can get to the orthographic-morphemic stage without first having mastered the alphabetic-phonemic stage (Gough and Tunmer, 1986). But studies show that there are readers who have acquired good orthographic ability despite having a persistent phonological deficit (Seymour and Elder, 1992). Moreover, we have also shown that the variation in reading ability among dyslexic eighth-graders was determined primarily by the variation in their ability to read orthographically, while the variation in reading ability among our normal eighth-graders was determined mainly by their phonological skills (Bjaalid, Høien and Lundberg, 1995). These findings lend support to the notion that dyslexics can, if given enough time, acquire good orthographic decoding skills even though they cannot directly overcome their phonological deficit (Fawcett and Nicolson, 1995).

Nonetheless, we still maintain that really well-specified orthographic identities seem to be the privilege of those who have a good phonological ability. The orthographic reading we seen in 'well-compensated' dyslexics is often found to be a word recognition process build on incomplete letter information. Therefore, the contextual cues function as an important supplement for their correct decoding. In situations that make greater demands on their orthographic strategy, for example when reading words only presented for a brief moment on a computer screen, their number of errors increases. They have learned to master reading, but the major problem for compensated dyslexics with a lack of well-specified orthographic identities is the great number of spelling errors they make.

Phonological Difficulties: Delayed Maturation or a Specific Deficit?

There is a great amount of variation in *the age* at which pupils achieve their maximum level of ability (their plateau), and *how high* a degree of ability they achieve.

A common topic of discussion is whether reading problems can be viewed as a part of a pupil's generally delayed maturation, or whether they are due to a deficit in one or more cognitive-linguistic abilities.

The *delayed maturation theory* claims that the poor reader will sooner or later catch up; it is just a question of time. The *deficit theory*, on the other hand, claims that the poor reader lacks an essential ability-a wound time alone will not heal.

The way to decide this question is through *longitudinal studies*, that is, studies that follow the same group of readers for many years and measure their reading ability at several intervals. Very few longitudinal studies have been carried out. Most studies of skilled and unskilled readers are what we call *cross section studies*; studies that take a 'snapshot' of how well a group of readers are doing at one point in time. To add to the problem, many of these cross section studies use different reading tests; this makes it difficult to compare the findings from one studies to another. There is, however, one good longitudinal study which has controlled for most of the problems that have pointed out in earlier longitudinal studies. In The Connecticut Longitudinal Study (Francis et al., 1996), children were followed over a nine-year period starting in preschool. The results from this study do not lend support to the delayed maturation theory. The poor readers in Connecticut achieved their highest level of reading ability at the same age as their normal-reading cohorts (at age 11 or 12), but the difference in reading ability between the good and the poor readers was the same then as it was in the third grade four or five years before. We should also note that there was not any difference in reading development in readers with 'specific reading difficulty' as opposed to those with 'general reading difficulty.'

Francis et al. claim that their data are most in line with the deficit theory. Pupils who read poorly, no matter which definition was used, all function poorly on tasks that make demands on their phonological awareness, for example when they are asked to divide a word into its constituent phonemes. This deficit in the phonological area can be measured even before the child starts school, and repeated tests can track the child's development through time. One test alone does not provide enough basis for diagnosing the child has having a 'phonological deficit,' because there are individual variations in the age at which child reach their plateau. The point is to make several measurements in order to ascertain whether the child's reading development halts before the child reaches the level of phonological ability needed to become a skilled reader.

In another longitudinal study, Jacobson and Lundberg (in print) followed 93 reading-challenged children from second to ninth grade. Most of them (79 pupils) never achieved normal reading ability. Only 14 pupils were able to overcome their reading problems. This study gives indirect support to the deficit theory. But some of their pupils, albeit only a few, showed a reading development more in line with the delayed maturation theory.

Problems in Automatization

A skill is usually deemed automatic when it is rapid, does not make great demands on processing capacity, takes place beyond conscious control, and when it includes parallel processing (Fawcett and Nicolson, 1994; Yap and van der Leij, 1994a, 1994b). Automatic word decoding is characterized as the correct and rapid reading of words (Samuels, 1985). Dyslexia is the opposite. Poorly automated word decoding is most clearly seen during the reading of words in isolation (Yap and van der Leij, 1994a, 1994b). When these readers read a well-connected text, their word decoding improves, probably because they are able to draw upon contextual clues

In addition to presenting words in isolation, another way of revealing poor decoding ability is to limit the amount of time the reader has available for decoding. This is very easily done on a personal computer. Here various exposure times can be selected as part of the experiment. If we compare the decoding results of pupils on words presented on the screen for five seconds with their results on words presented for one-fifth of a second, we find that readers with a highly automatic decoding skill score pretty much the same at both speeds. But the dyslexics score much worse on the briefly presented words than on the words they are given time to think about. Their decoding is not automatic. Studies carried out by Yap and van der Leij (1994) also show that dyslexics can improve their decoding ability by training on briefly presented words. This training effect has a positive transference to real-life text-reading.

An interesting question here is whether poor readers' lack of automaticity in word decoding is symptomatic of some general problem in achieving automaticity in other skills. Fawcett and Nicolson (1994) have formulated the 'Automaticity deficit hypothesis.' They see the difficulties in word decoding as a result of a phonological deficit and a deficient ability to achieve automaticity in other skills such as throwing a ball, tying one's shoelaces, walking backwards, copying figures, and balancing on one foot. They found statistically significant differences in how well dyslexics performed on these task as compared to reading-matched younger children.

Handwriting and articulation are also motoric skills, and studies show that dyslexic children are less skilled at these activities than are younger reading-matched children (Stanovich, 1988; Søvik et al., 1996).

When pupils are asked to perform a task, e.g. word decoding, that they have not learned to do automatically, they have to draw upon cognitive resources. This causes fatigue, and can explain the tiredness and inattention which also characterize these pupils.

Brief Summary

We have now examined the different strategies and processes that word decoding builds on. Two decoding strategies are of particular importance: the phonological and the orthographic strategy. Each of the strategies employs a unique set of psychological processes. Dyslexia is characterized by a deficit in one or more decoding strategies, and this deficit can be traced back to a deficit in one or more of the underlying psychological processes. The principle on which a process-analytic diagnostic practice is founded is that a pupil's ability to perform various types of reading tasks will tell us which of his or her underlying processes are normal and which are not functioning optimally. Through administering a series of tests we are able to draw a reading profile for a pupil which takes into consideration both quantitative and qualitative aspects of his or her unique reading ability. How this is done will be the topic of Chapter 7. But first we will need to look at spelling difficulties, the topic in the next chapter. Along with decoding difficulties, spelling problems are a characteristic feature of dyslexia.

CHAPTER 3

SPELLING DIFFICULTY: A MAJOR SYMPTOM OF DYSLEXIA

Compared to the amount of research done on reading, surprisingly little work has been done on the psychology of how we write. And most of the work done on the writing process has been limited to spelling. Researchers have looked at the strategies one uses in order to spell a word correctly, and much of the work has focused on the spelling errors young writers make, in order to gain insight into the underlying causal factors of the poor spelling. Most commonly, researchers have looked at how well writers spell words in isolation, that is, when the words are dictated in a test, not in the pupils' own written work (Boder, 1973; Gjessing, 1977).

More recently it has become common to focus on the writing process itself (for overview, see Berninger, 1994, 1995). The writing process involves much more than merely spelling words correctly. It includes such skills as composing sentences, paragraphs and texts. The writer is supposed to give clear expression to his or her thoughts via the medium of written words and sentences (for overview, see Levy and Ransdell, 1996).

In order to help students learn to write, teachers need to know about the writing process. They need to know about the perceptual and motor aspects of writing (Kao, Galen and van Hoosain, 1986), and about process-oriented writing exercises. In this chapter we will not deal with the teaching aspects of process-oriented writing, but instead refer the reader to the rich literature on the subject In this chapter we will focus on the spelling process and on the various strategies writers use to figure out how to spell a word.

Correct spelling, of course, is not the point of learning to write. Nonetheless, spelling is important for several reasons. First of all, schools have traditionally emphasized good spelling, and students are expected to learn a whole series of spelling rules of increasing complexity. One reason schools have put so much emphasis on correct spelling is that writing is visible and permanent. Misspelled words stick out, and, at least for the adult writer, they are odious, leading the reader to assume (perhaps wrongly) that the writer 'doesn't know what he's talking about.' Obviously, dyslexic students suffer greatly because of such wide-spread attitudes. We will argue, in line with modern thinking, that schools should relax their demands for correct spelling. But we do believe that correct spelling is an important skill. As noted previously, we believe that reading and writing are closely connected skills, and that learning to do one of them helps the student learn to do the other. Teachers should be teaching both, pretty much at the same pace.

Another aspect of good spelling is that it necessary of achieving a good automaticity in writing. A student who struggles with spelling words correctly is a student who writes slowly and laboriously, with little joy. When the young student's mind is focused so strongly on this one aspect of writing, then he or she has little mental energy that can be devoted to other aspects of writing. The poor speller's writing proceeds at a snail's pace; thoughts the writer might have wanted to jot down vanish. A fluid speller, at a minimum, does not have this problem.

Stages in the Development of Spelling

Like reading skills, spelling skills develop according to various stages defined by which strategies the pupil uses (see e.g. Read, 1978). Early in the development, some spelling skills seem to develop before the corresponding reading skills; after that, spelling skills generally lag a bit behind reading skills.

Pseudo-spelling

As with reading, spelling, for most children, starts out with a stage of pseudo-writing. Long before children have learned any of the letters, they often pretend to write by filling pages with long, snaky lines of letter-like symbols. They can often 'read' these 'texts' in fanciful ways.

As the child's knowledge of the letters increases, this pretend-writing becomes more precise and considered. Many researchers have described in detail various aspects of pre-school children's pseudo-writing, and shown the importance of this stage for the child's subsequent development (see report by National Research Council, 1998).

Logographic-visual spelling

When children at the logographic stage of reading 'read,' say, the McDonald's logo, it is a recognition of a symbol that takes place without recourse to the alphabetic principle. They 'read' distinctive words just like they read pictures. If the characteristic M in the McDonald's logo is the tip-off when they 'read' it, then it will be prominently featured when they 'write' the word. At this stage, children's writing is more like drawing. They try to render the most salient aspects of a logo or sign, without giving the phonology of the word a thought. Sometimes a child will produce the first letter of a name or word correctly, but represent the rest of the word with a random assortment of letters and letter-like figures.

At this stage, children are very fond of writing their own names. They learn by copying an adult's writing, usually in capital letters. Some children get as far as being able to write a handful or so other words, with all the letters in the right order, yet still without using the alphabetic principle.

Alphabetic-phonemic spelling

This is when children begin to use the alphabetic principle. They analyze spoken words, picking out the phonemes, and then try to represent these with letters - usually capital letters. At the start of this phase, children often cannot read what they have written. (This is where their spelling skills outstrip their reading skills.) Read (1978) and Chomsky (1970) have described how preschoolers spontaneously invent their own perfectly logical, but utterly nonconventional, spelling systems to represent the sounds of words.

As their reading ability increases, children get better at analyzing the sounds of the words they want to write, and they do a better job of segmenting words into phonemes. They generally spell words 'regularly,' i.e. according to the simplest, most basic rules of spelling - one letter for one phoneme - not caring about the finer points of silent letters or digraphs like *ph*. Sometimes their phonetic analyses show a remarkable degree of sophistication. A child who writes the name of his dog Spot as *SBOT* is a child who has latched on to a non-functional, subphonemic feature of English phonology only trained linguists are used to noticing: i.e. that the letter *p* in the combination *sp-* is pronounced with a sound quite like /b/. What the child hasn't learned, but surely will gain awareness of in due time, is that English spelling-rules, as opposed to say Italian or Spanish, just do not allow for words to begin with *sb-*. Words beginning with *sb-* violate the orthotactic rules of English.

Perhaps the high degree of phonological sensitivity children at this stage show is related to their often-noted ability to pick up new dialects and even languages without accents. In this regard, dyslexic children seem to have no handicap: if they move to another part of the country, or to a foreign country where they hear a new language, they can acquire the local pronunciation as quickly as normal-reading children in similar circumstances. Children in general are clever at hearing and imitating the sounds of a language, but dyslexic children - for reasons we don't yet understand - seem to be less able to break a word down into its component phonemes. Analyzing a word phonemically is a very abstract process. It involves being able to sort out the myriad of sounds heard in spoken English into a very limited number of higher order, abstract units, the 40 or so phonemes. This appears to be a much more complicated or abstract task than analyzing a word phonetically.

At this stage, too, children begin to understand some of the complexities of writing, namely that one and the same phoneme can be represented in more than one way in written language, and that one and the same letter or combination of letters can be used to represent different sounds. The sound /aj/ can be spelled *I* or *eye*, or it can be represented by *-i* (in the word *hi*), by *-ie* (as in *tie*), *-igh* (*high*), *-y* (*my*) and so on. Similarly, the letter *u* can be used to represent many different vowel-sounds: *you, butcher, but, mute, pull, though*, etc. Moreover, at this stage children begin to develop a feeling for which combinations of letters are very common, and which are rare. Soon, the spelling *SBOT* will seem strange to them, too.

Because writing never really can represent the sounds of spoken language very well, no one can write like they speak. Even in educated speech, sounds get slurred together, reduced, assimilated, elided, clipped, and left out. Even people who attend closely to the niceties of pronunciation leave out the *d* in *good morning*, usually reducing it to an *m* (*gummorning*). There is nothing sloppy about this; this is just the way spoken language works. We speak with a high degree of what is known as *co-articulation*: we don't produce the string of phonemes one at a time as discrete units, but link them together in a blurred, smeared chain. Just about any given sound in a segment of speech will usually be altered by the quality of the sounds coming before and after it. To grasp the idea, say the words *hip* and *hop* aloud, and listen to the *h*-sounds. In both cases the phoneme /h/ is colored by the vowel coming after it. It is as if the speech-organs anticipate what is coming, and act accordingly, the goal being smooth, fluid speech.

There is nothing mystical about the principle of co-articulation. It is how our muscles usually react. For example, say you want to pick up a pen on the desk in front of you. You don't first move your arm so that your hand is positioned above the pen, and then move your fingers into a grasping position. That would look like a poorly designed robot. What you do instead is this: Almost at the same time as you start moving your arm, your hand starts getting into the appropriate position for picking up the pen. Your motions are fluid and co-articulated, because you know what you are going to do after your hand comes into position over the pen. You are going to pick it up.

Now, one could, in theory, design an alphabetical system that reflected all the subtle changes that phonemes go through as they pass the organs of speech. But such a system would be immensely impractical and impossible for people other than trained linguists to learn. So, the alphabetical systems of our languages simplify the phonology to a high degree. Because we know we're talking about a *good* morning, we write out the word *good*, even though the *d* is silent in this instance, thereby preserving for the reader the meaning of the utterance. Because we know (albeit only on some tacit level of awareness) that *h*'s get colored by the vowels coming after them, we don't need to represent this fact in writing. Why would we want a dozen or so different symbols for what we perceive as the same phoneme with different phonological colorings? Alphabetical writing systems simplify phonology by seeking to represent spoken phenomena at a higher level of abstraction than mere sounds, namely the level of phonemes - the abstract 'things' that remain when you take out the particulars of the situation such as phonological context, dialectical variation, idiosyncratic pronunciations, etc. This is why writing is never a straightforward process of simply encoding what you hear. And it is one of the main reasons that writing, unlike talking, has to be taught and learned. And it is writing's abstract nature that seems to be the stumbling block for dyslexic children.

Sometimes children at the alphabetic-phonemic stage of spelling write only parts of words. *Coffee* can be represented as *KF*, *house* as *HS*, *tomatoes* as *TMTS*. As we see, it is mainly vowels that get left out. Consonants carry more information and are less ambiguous, so young writers latch onto them more easily. Sometimes the children let the *name* of the letter supply the intended vowel-sound: *are* gets spelled *R*, *you U, begin BGIN*, and *Emily MLE*. A similar process of reduction seems to be taking place when the child writes *techr* for *teacher* or *frnd* for friend.

When a child writes *SBIL* for *spill*, or *SDOR* for *store*, it looks as if he or she is unable to properly analyze the sound of the intended word. But, as with the dog named *SBOT*, this is far from the case. These errors prove unambiguously that the child is indeed working with the sounds, not copying the word as a visual pattern from a workbook. These are good misspellings; they tell us the child is working in the right way. In both of these cases, the child has substituted a voiced consonant for its unvoiced 'twin' after the initial letter *s*. *SBIL* is wrong, we think, because the letter *B* is how we encode the voiced consonant /b/, not the correct unvoiced consonant /p/. And the same with *SDOR*: The *D* is wrong because we hear the unvoiced consonant /t/.

Or do we? Phoneticians have fairly recently carried out experiments to isolate exactly what it is we think we hear. Using modern recording devices they systematically altered the length of the *s*-sound in words like these, and they found out that they could get the consonant following the *s* to change character simply by tweaking the length of the *s*-sound a few milliseconds: *t*'s suddenly got perceived as *d*'s and *b*'s turned into *p*'s. The problem with spellings like *SBIL* and *SDOR* is not that they are 'unphonetical,' because they in fact are *very* phonetical; but simply that they look very strange - to the experienced reader (who has intuitively grasped the orthotactic rules). If you try to pronounce them, you'll find that they are actually good representations of how we say *spill* and *store*. In fact, *SBIL* is in at least one way *better* than the conventionally mandated spelling *spill*. The /p/ in this word is unaspirated, that it, it lacks the little puff of air we usually make when we pronounce the sounds that we encode with the letter *p*. To hear the aspiration, say *pill* and *bill*. Part of the difference is the voicing of the /b/, and part of the difference is the aspiration of the /p/. When the initial *s*-sound confuses our perception of the voiced/unvoiced distinction of the consonant that follows, and the aspiration of the /p/ is missing, *SBIL* becomes a very phonetical spelling indeed. When children make these errors, it is not because they don't analyze the sounds properly, but simply because they haven't seen the words enough times for the correct spellings to sink in.

Alphabetic-phonemic spelling shows that the young writer is using a *phonological strategy for spelling,* and that is a great step forward.

Orthographic-morphemic spelling

At this stage children begin to approach the conventionally correct and assured spelling of adults. They can write a large number of words without having to think too much about them. Not only are they able to encode strings of phonemes successfully, but they even begin to take into consideration the *morphemes* of language as well. Morphemes, we remember, are prefixes, suffixes, and word-stems - the parts of words at an even higher level of abstraction than letters or phonemes. While our alphabetical languages generally encode phonemes with letters (however imperfectly), they also try to retain the spelling of morphemes even though they get pronounced with different phonemes in different contexts. For example: listen to the phonemes of the words *grade* and *gradual*, or *nation* and *national*. In both cases the vowel of the word-stem changes from one phoneme to another when we stick on the adjectival suffix. This change in pronunciation of the word-stems *could* have been encoded in the spellings; indeed, that would have the advantage of making the spellings more 'regular' or more 'phonetic.' But it is a good thing that English (usually) keeps the spelling of word-stems constant, because then we can see the semantic relationship between the word-stem and derived form: *Gradual* and *national* come from, and are the adjective forms of, the nouns *grade* and *nation*. The unchanged spellings make this obvious.

The pervasive morphemic *-ed* suffix for denoting simple past tense of most verbs is another example. Phonetically, these verbs end in a variety of phonemes: /ed/, /id/, /t/, and so on. Instead of encoding these sounds in a variety of ways, our spelling system lets them all end in *-ed*, thus helping us see them as past tense verbs. Phonemic spelling is nice, but the point of reading is to understand the text, not to pronounce it, and having a morphemic component in English spelling gets readers more quickly to the meaning than a purely phonemic spelling system would (Elbro, 1990; Elbro and Arnbak, 1996).

At this stage of the child's learning to spell, the orthographic representations of words in the child's mental dictionary are well established, and the child has acquired a lot of knowledge about morphemes. Dyslexics only very rarely achieve this level of proficiency (Bruck, 1988, 1990).

Types of Spelling Errors

A misspelled word is not always a sign of a pupil's inadequacy. It is more productive for the teacher to look upon the error as an interesting sign of the child's efforts at solving the problem, in particular a sign of his choice of strategy. Dyslexic children often have a lot of errors in their written work, and their errors show a high degree of instability. For example, we can often find the same word spelled in different ways in the same text. Especially for dyslexic students, we must not draw hasty conclusions on the basis of only a few errors. We need to try to find their pattern of errors, the kinds of mistakes that appear again and again in their work.

When we analyze spelling errors we need to keep in mind the difference between *errors of knowledge* and *errors of performance*. Errors of knowledge are the mistakes a pupil makes because he or she doesn't know better. Errors in performance are slips of the pen; the student knows how to spell the word correctly, but didn't.

Errors of knowledge

When the writer doesn't remember how a particular word is spelled, then he or she has to try to sound it out. This is the phonological strategy. When we use this strategy we often wind up with a spelling that represents the pronunciation of the word correctly, but which is conventionally wrong. Examples would be spelling *mice* as *mise* or *house* as *howse*. Irregularly spelled words, that is words which don't follow the usual rules, often get regularized. An example would be *women*, which could be written as *wimen*. Errors like *mise, howse,* and *wimen* are what we call *orthographical errors,* because these misspellings break orthographic rules, but not phonological rules.

Phonological errors, on the other hand, are misspellings that yield phonologically wrong sounds when you read them. Spelling *fast* as *fact* would be a phonological error. As we have pointed out, it is not always easy to be sure that a misspelled word is phonologically wrong. Writing *school* as *sgule* looks absurd, but actually sounds right when you read it. And we have to be familiar with the pupil's dialect. A child who has just moved from Boston may well write *Daddy pakt the ca* (Daddy parked the car) without this being a *phonological* error - for him. Because of his dialect background, he won't readily 'hear' the *r*'s in words like *parked* and *car.* (And nobody hears a *d* in *parked.*) Often we find some bits of correct orthographic knowledge in these mistakes. For example, the child who misspelled *fast* as *fact* most likely had a correct image of the word as being about four letters long, starting with an *f*, having *a* as vowel and ending in an *t*. It was just the easily confused pair of letters *s-c* that caused the misspelling.

Specific deviation from rules of writing are what we call errors such as lack of capitalization (*i* for *I*), mistakes in punctuation, incorrectly formed letters (such as backward *s*'es) and mistakes with compound words (*police man* or *schoolpencils*).

Reversal errors are mistakes in the order of the letters. Writing *from* as *form* or *boat* as *baot* would be examples here. They are technically termed *incomplete reversals.* Sometimes we find complete reversals, such as *nus* for *sun.*

Errors in performance

These are the mistakes we make when we are not thinking, tired, frustrated, etc. Many reversals, for example, are due to a poor performance, not to a lack of knowledge. Another typical performance error is leaving out a letter that has already been written once, e.g. *t-shirs* for *t-shirts,* or *missing perons* for *missing persons.*

Analysis of Errors

We will look briefly at two different approaches to the analysis of spelling errors. Wiggen (1990) analyzed the spelling errors in nearly 1,000 student texts (open-ended homework assignments). These were written by approx. 700 pupils from grades two through six in Norway. The results showed that age, sex, and socio-linguistic factors were the variables that explained most of the errors. (Wiggen also found a confusion between the two forms of written Norwegian to be a factor.) The number of errors diminished through the years of schooling, and boys consistently had more errors than girls. On average, about every third word in the second-grade texts was misspelled, as opposed to about every tenth word in grade six. But there were huge individual differences among the pupils.

One of Wiggen's most interesting findings was that about half of all the errors were specific deviations from the rules of writing: punctuation mistakes, compounding errors, and the like. When he looked at the types of spelling mistakes that were occurring, he found more errors with consonants than with vowels. Consonant errors were often errors of omission, while vowel errors were usually due to the pupil choosing the wrong vowel to represent the vowel-sound.

Bråten (1990) has developed four categories of words that can help us sort out the kinds of spelling errors young writers can commit. He divided words into four categories, E-words, R-words, M-words, and U-words.

E-words are the phonetically *Easy* words, which are spelled with a simple, one-to-one correspondence between phonemes and graphemes. An example of an E-word would be *hat*. There is not much doubt as to how it is written, although some young writers might put an extra *t* at the end. R-words are also 'Regular,' but the rules they follow are more complex. *Hate* is such a word. Its spelling is quite regular, but the pupil has to understand how the silent *e* at the end changes the vowel-sound in the middle. At first children learn these words one at a time, without understanding the underlying rule. But when they do grasp the rule, they tend to overgeneralize, producing such interesting mistakes as *bate* (for *bait*) and *rale* (for *rail*).

Bråten's M-words are those words that make demands on the pupil's *Morphemic* knowledge. An example here would be *rode*, the past tense of *to ride*. Phonetically, we could spell the word *road* or *rowed*, but we don't, because we know (intuitively) that our spelling system seeks to preserve morphemes; *rode* is the correct spelling because it is analogous to *ride*, while *rowed* is obviously the past tense of *to row* and *road* must be something else entirely. Another example is *wrote*, not *rote*, again because of the analogy with *write*. Children typically start out trying to figure out the spellings of M-words by applying the phonetical rules they have learned. Only later do they make the morphological connection and get them right. These words make demands not only on the child's understanding of how the sounds of language can be encoded in letters, but on how language itself works, and children with major spelling problems such as dyslexics do not seem to spontaneously grasp the morphological principle (Elbro, 1990). They also seem to attack these problem words in nonproductive ways (Bråten, 1990).

Finally, the U-words are those with the truly *Unique* spellings, the ones you can't sound out. These include both foreign names and words (*Nike* and *Des Moines*) as well as some very highly frequent words that defy sounding out (*women, people, have, said, give, of*). These words make demands on the reader's memory for what words look like; the phonological strategy doesn't get them beyond the first letter or two, nor does morphemic knowledge help much.

Spelling and Speaking

There is broad evidence that writers usually try to spell words they are not familiar with on the basis of how they sound. Their phonological analysis is usually articulatory: Children may say the word aloud or just mouth the word with their tongue and lips. The consonants have comparatively unambiguous articulatory identities: tongues flap and lips pucker in ways that are relatively easy to identify. Vowels, on the other hand, are crucially dependent on very precise positioning of the tongue. The difference in tongue position during the vowel-sounds in, say, *Jim's* and *James* is very small.

It is obvious then that spoken language plays a large role in spelling. The new words that generally cause the most problems are those that deviate the most from the rules, or, to put it more precisely, that follow the more obscure rules. But here we have to remember that a word one child thinks is very regular, may be irregular to another child from another part of the country (Desberg et al., 1980). Wiggen (1990) has also documented that moving from one dialect region to another during elementary school can confuse the pupil and disturb the foundation for his learning to read and write.

Spelling and Reading

In general we can say that the reading difficulties we find with dyslexic students always are accompanied by spelling difficulties. Moreover, research has shown that spelling difficulties are more resistant to remediation than reading problems are. Well-tailored remedial programmes can help many dyslexics to read better, but their spelling problems unfortunately often persist. Therefore, the gap between their reading and spelling abilities increases with age (Bruck, 1990).

Spelling includes many subprocesses, involving phonological, morphological, semantic and orthographic skills. The fact that some skilled readers also are poor spellers shows that reading and spelling to a certain degree are independent skills. For most people, however, the two skills correlate well (Søvik, Heggberget, & Samuelstuen, 1996).

The difference between the two skills, of course, is that reading is decoding letters into sounds well enough to arrive at the phonological identity of the word, while spelling a word correctly entails encoding the sounds into letters in accordance with the right rule. The processes are not symmetrical. Confronted with these three letter-strings: *road, rode,* and *rowed*, the *reader* arrives in each case at the correct pronunciation: /rod/. But when the *speller* wants to write one of them, he needs something more in order to spell it right, e.g. a feeling for morphemes or a good memory for orthography.

We often use different strategies when reading a word and when spelling it. Early in the first grade we often find children who read words logographically, but spell them phonetically. Somewhat older students will often read orthographically but still spell phonetically. These differences in reading and spelling strategies can often be explained by the developmental stages of spelling and reading, but sometimes they are due to the lack of symmetry between the two tasks.

Spelling phonologically entails hearing or imagining the sound of the word, and then pulling the sounds apart into separate phonemes. This is called *phonological analysis*. Reading phonologically, on the other hand, entails saying aloud or imagining the string of phonemes the letters seem to be representing, and then sticking them together to make a word. This is called *phonological synthesis*. Generally the analysis is easier to do and is acquired earlier than the synthesis, so we often find children who can encode a nonword correctly, but who can't yet read the same string of letters. But with some children it is the other way around: they can decode a given letter-string, yet are unable to spell the same word in a plausible way (Bryant and Bradley, 1980).

The writer can also check his spelling by writing the word down to see whether it looks right. Orthographic word-recognition, as it is called, is not always a reliable method. If it were, then it would be the case that those readers who are good at orthographic reading would always be good at spelling, but that is not the case. As mentioned before, there are many skilled readers who spell very poorly. Nonetheless, visual checking of spelling does help most spellers somewhat (Shuren, Maher and Heilman, 1996).

Spelling Errors and the Definition of Dyslexia

According to our definition, dyslexia is a condition caused by a deficit in phonological skills. In order to read and write, pupils have to become conscious of the fact that words are constructed of phonemes. Dyslexics do poorly on tests that measure skills in manipulating phonemes. Poor spellers do poorly on the same tests (Goswami and Bryant, 1990).

Our hypothesis is that incomplete phonological representations of words in the child's mental lexicon and the child's poor phonemic awareness make the spelling process difficult for these children. When, for instance, the second *u* in *usual* often doesn't get pronounced, then it won't easily stick in the memory. This is why dyslexics often leave out letters that are silent or not fully sounded, spelling *usual* as *usal* or *uzul*, or *error* as *err* or *ar*. In a study by Bruck and Treiman (1990), they found that poor spellers also scored poorly on tests of phonemic awareness. It appears that writing, to an even greater degree than reading, depends on specifically phonological skills.

In our opinion, the underlying problem with dyslexia, the phonological deficit, can explain most of the decoding and spelling problems we see in dyslexic children. If their phonological deficit is indeed the culprit, then we should expect to see a greater percentage of purely phonological spelling mistakes among the dyslexics' errors than we find among normal readers. Yet research has not always borne this out (Bailet, 1990; Moats, 1993; Worthy and Invernizzi, 1990). On the contrary, analysis of the types of errors has shown that fully 70 to 80 percent of the dyslexics' misspellings yield phonetically correct words (Moats, 1993). How can this be explained?

Moats (1996) claims that much of the earlier research done on types of spelling errors was lacking in precision. The categories traditionally used to classify the errors were not sensitive enough to catch the phonological spelling difficulties. Moats studied 19 boys (ages 14 to 17 years), all of whom had major spelling problems. They received a sound remedial programme that went over two years. She studied their progress and performed a thorough analysis of their spelling errors. Her analysis was based on three categories of errors: Phonological errors (letter-strings that couldn't be pronounced like the target word), morphophonemic errors (letter-strings that broke with the morphological conventions, such as *slapt* for *slapped*), and orthographic errors (letter-strings that could be pronounced like the target word, but that were conventionally wrong, e.g. *tode* for *toad*). Of the 19 boys, 10 didn't show much progress in the course of the two years. An analysis of these 10 subjects' spelling errors revealed many phonological errors: they neglected to represent some sounds, they added letters that weren't in the pronunciation of the target word, they made substitutions, etc. These results support the notion that the problem underlying dyslexia is a lack of sensitivity for phonological and morphological structures.

Moats' results are supported by a study done by Worthy and Vise (1996). They compared the spelling errors of adult dyslexics with the errors seen in a control group of young people without dyslexia, but who had the same general ability to spell words as the adult dyslexics. The two groups showed no difference in the number of reversals, and the dyslexics had a somewhat better orthographic memory than the controls. But the really interesting finding was that the dyslexics had a number of phonological and morphological errors of the type only rarely found among the controls. These results support Moats' contention that the spelling difficulties dyslexics have are associated with a specific deficit in their ability to perform phonological and morphophonological analyses.

We know that young children develop phonological skills gradually. Some phonemes and some consonant-clusters are harder to articulate than others. These difficulties in articulation include elisions, additions, and substitutions. Typically, young children will have a problem pronouncing all the consonants in complicated clusters (pronouncing *sprite* like *spite*) and in getting the voiced-unvoiced distinction right in single consonants (confusing *b*'s with *p*'s or *t*'s with *d*'s, and so on). The same pattern of error turns up in the dyslexics' spelling (Read, 1996; Treiman, 1993, 1997). The spelling process has the additional difficulty caused by co-articulation. Smearing the sounds together, as we do even in careful speech, makes it hard to pick out and identify the individual phonemes. Another matter is that dyslexics have very little feeling for morphemes, especially word-stems and suffixes, because they don't read very much.

A deficiency in segmenting and identifying phonemes hinders the pupil in encoding them in letters when spelling, and in retrieval word elements that are not very well defined in speech. This deficiency in phonological ability will therefore delay the acquisition of a well-stocked orthographic memory - the storehouse of words that can be recognized on sight. If it were possible for the orthographic memory to be built up in spite of the pupil's phonological deficit, then poor spellers would at least be learning how to spell the highly frequent words. Moats claims that this is unfortunately not happening. Her findings indicate on the contrary that phonological ability and orthographic memory go hand in hand. For her group of dyslexic boys, the boys with the fewest phonological misspellings also had the best orthographic memories, and the boys with the most phonological misspellings also had the weakest orthographic memories. These findings indicate that phonological ability is important to the acquisition of a good orthographic memory.

Furthermore, Moats found that the phonological substitutions her spellers made were not random. Usually, when they chose the wrong letter to represent a phoneme, they substituted a close relative, that is, a letter that represented a phoneme that we articulate nearly the same as the phoneme they were supposed to represent. For example, misspelling *very* as *fery* misrepresents the /v/ with the letter *f*. But *v*'s and *f*'s are articulated almost the same, the only difference being that /v/ is voiced and /f/ is not. This shows the close relationship between phonology and articulation. In a sense, we 'write with our tongues'. We see this happen when we look at young children writing or spelling. They focus on the sounds of the words by moving their tongues and lips. This unvoiced sounding out may be the reason that they often mix up voiced and unvoiced consonants, i.e *d*'s and *t*'s, *z*'s and *s*'s, *b*'s and *p*'s, and so on.

In reading research a relatively modern approach is to use control groups that match the study group in level of ability (see Chapter 1). When we analyze spelling errors we find it interesting to compare dyslexics with younger, normal pupils at the same level of general ability; i.e. pupils a few grades below who make about the same number of spelling errors as the group we are studying. The difference in types of errors we then find between the two groups can give us some indication as to the nature of the problem the dyslexic spellers have. Results of level-matched studies have shown that the older dyslexics had better developed orthographic memories and weaker phonological abilities than their younger, normal counterparts (Pennington et al., 1986).

Good spelling ability depends crucially on awareness of morphemes and grammar. In order to spell well, a child has to have some understanding of how words change form according to their grammatical function. When we are talking about someone who was in a rowboat yesterday, then we write *The man rowed*, not *rode* or *road*. A child can only do this right when he or she is aware of two things: the first being the grammar of the sentence; here, that the verb is in the simple past tense. Secondly, the child needs to know that the *d* we hear in the word is the familiar morpheme, the *-ed* suffix we add to verbs to make them past tense. Being aware of these two things is called *morphosyntactical awareness*.

Spelling Errors and Subgroups of Dyslexia

Within the field there has been much discussion of whether or not an analysis of the types of spelling errors can lead to a better diagnostic practice of dyslexia. Even though there are those who feel that spelling errors can help us group dyslexics better (Boder, 1973; Gjessing, 1977; Snowling, 1981), most researchers do not (Bruck, 1988; Worthy and Invernizzi, 1990).

Gjessing and Boder carried out qualitative analyses of both reading errors and spelling errors by subgrouping dyslexics as either auditive dyslexics (dysphonetic dyslexia), visual dyslexics (dyseidetic dyslexia) and auditive-visual dyslexics.

When looking at spelling, they claimed that the auditive dyslexics are characterized by a lot of phonological misspellings, while the visual dyslexics are characterized by their frequent orthographic misspellings. As we would suspect, the auditive-visual dyslexics had more of a mix of types of errors. Furthermore, the three subgroups also make the same characteristic types of errors when reading. Boder (1971) claimed that 70 percent of his dyslexics were auditive dyslexics.

Letter-reversals have been focused on in the research. This type of error was traditionally considered a 'sure sign' of a failing child's dyslexia. Furthermore, the incomplete reversals (*form* for *from*) were often thought to be definitive of a special type of dyslexia, namely auditive dyslexia, while the complete reversals (*nus* for *sun*) were thought to be indicative of visual dyslexia (Gjessing, 1977; Boder and Jarrico, 1984).

It is questionable, however, whether or not reversals should be given any special attention when diagnosing dyslexia (Moats, 1993; Pennington et al., 1986). Wiggen (1992), working with Norwegian children, has shown that reversals are quite rare, and that when they do occur, they usually can be explained by the speller's dialect, or as a result of influence from other norms of language, either written or oral.

In serious cases of spelling difficulty, we believe that a thorough analysis of the errors will reveal an overweight of phonological and morphological errors (Moats, 1996). But, again, we have to emphasize that it is no easy task to perform a thorough analysis. The task demands a profound knowledge of phonology and linguistics. Wiggen's results show how complicated this work is.

Despite the fact that we have been emphasizing the importance of phonological skills for the acquisition of good spelling ability, we must point out that there is some evidence that orthographic identities of words can be acquired even though the student's phonological system functions very poorly. In these cases, we assume that the student has acquired his orthographic identities by using strategies that explicitly draw his attention to the how words are spelled (Berninger, 1994; Henry, 1988).

Handwriting

Many dyslexic pupils have poorer handwriting than other pupils. Dysgraphia, Latin for 'problem with writing,' is the term we use for those who have a major problem with penmanship. One cause of the condition could be the delayed development of fine motor-skills that characterize many dyslexic children (Søvik and Arntzen, 1992; Søvik, Arntzen and Karlsdottir, 1993). But an emotional component may also be at work. Dyslexic children don't like letters. For them, they carry a negative emotional charge; letters are things to be avoided. And because the dyslexic child may well have succeeded in avoiding writing exercises, he or she may have had less practice. This too adds to the penmanship problem. Finally, some young writers who are unsure of how to spell a word write it sloppily, hoping that the teacher will 'read' the garbled word in the correct way.

Cicci (1983) tells of several types of handwriting problems that often accompany dyslexia: inappropriate grip on the pen, overly tense grip, wrong positioning of the words on the page, inappropriate size of letters and spaces, slow writing tempo, and poor coordination. When we are confronted by all or most of these problems, we are tempted to give up: to just let these children write any way they want. But there is a good argument for working with the child to improve penmanship: learning to form the letters well provides the young writer with kinesthetic feedback. Not only does the child learn to see what well-formed letters look like, but he or she gets to feel what it feels like to make them.

In several studies, Søvik and his co-workers have looked at the associations between reading, spelling, and penmanship (Søvik, Arntzen and Samuelstuen, 1993; Søvik, Heggberget and Samuelstuen, 1996; Søvik et al., 1996;). They found a strong correlation among these skills. They have also compared the developmental pattern and level of achievement of three groups: normal readers, dyslexic children and dysgraphic children. These studies showed that normal readers were more skilled than the other two groups at writing legibly and in attaining a good speed of writing and a good rhythm. Dyslexic children as a group wrote slower than both the normal-readers and the dysgraphics. In measures of legibility and rhythm, the dysgraphic children scored significantly poorer than the others. Moreover, these studies also showed pretty much the same developmental curves in handwriting for normal-readers and children with handwriting problems, and they pointed out the good effect children's own exercises in writing have during the first three or four years of schooling. These exercises can help hinder the development of dysgraphia.

Karlsdottir (1996a, b, c) has carried out longitudinal studies to examine the effect of choice of script in first grade - block letters or cursive - on reading and writing ability in later grades. Approx. 100 pupils were taught to write block letters in first grade, and about the same number were taught to use cursive script right from the start. From the second grade on all pupils were taught to write cursive. She followed all the subjects until grade five, when she checked both qualitative and quantitative aspects of their handwriting and their reading and spelling abilities. She did not find significant differences between the two groups in regard to writing speed, penmanship, reading ability or spelling ability. But as she points out, it is still an open question whether choice of script might be important for *dyslexic* students.

Teachers probably tend to give lower grades to written work with bad handwriting. For some people with major handwriting problems, personal computers are a boon. But children still need to learn good penmanship. Handwriting is a skill people will need their whole lives, and very poor handwriting, like poor spelling, will often be taken as a sign of stupidity. In the higher grades, however, computers can be of great help for students with writing problems, especially when they master the use of spelling-checkers.

Spelling Strategies

As with reading, there are several different strategies one can use to *spell* words, and the two most important are the phonological and the orthographic strategies.

When we use the phonological strategy, we break the word down into its constituent phonemes, which we then encode in graphemes. This encoding is done on the basis of the *phoneme-grapheme correspondence rules*. In a language with a perfectly regular orthography, where there is a strict correspondence between phonemes and graphemes, this strategy alone would ensure that we could spell all words and nonwords correctly. But except for a few minor languages which received their spelling-systems in modern times, e.g. Hawaiian, written languages are far from being perfectly phonetical. If Hawaiian, with its 12 phonemes which code smoothly into just 12 graphemes, is a speller's dream, then English (or French, for that matter) would have to be termed a nightmare. Generally speaking, the more complicated, overlapping, contradictory or inconsistent a language's phoneme-grapheme correspondence rules are, the more the speller just has to *know* how the word is spelled.

The orthographic strategy for spelling is this *knowing*. An experienced speller writes *people* correctly because he or she has learned how it is spelled. The orthographic representation of the sound of the word is remembered, and then retrieved when needed. The beauty of this strategy is that it permits the speller to spell correctly all the words he or she has learned, both regular, semi-regular, irregular, and unique words. The drawback of the orthographic strategy is that it gives the speller absolutely no help when he or she is trying to spell a new word, or (perhaps more frequently) when the speller has to choose among homophones like *rowed, road* and *rode* or *seeded, ceded,* and *seated,* or *utter* and *udder* or *latter* and *ladder* or (in many dialects) *Mary, marry,* and *merry.*

Shallice (1981) has given us a detailed description of an adult patient, P.R., who could read and spell normally, but who as a result of brain damage found it impossible to spell nonwords. P.R. had a deficit in the phonological spelling strategy, while his orthographic spelling strategy was intact. This form of agraphia is called *phonological agraphia.* A deficit in the phonological spelling strategy is thought primary to be caused by difficulties in performing phoneme segmentation. Several studies have shown that phoneme segmentation of spoken words is a complex task to learn to do (Liberman et al., 1980; Lundberg, 1984; Morais et al., 1979). Difficulties in segmenting phonemes show up as characteristic misspellings when the child is forced to use the phonological strategy. First and foremost we see a characteristic dropping of letters that are clearly pronounced in the word.

Beauvois and Derouesné (1981) have reported another adult patient with brain damage, G.R., with the opposite set of symptoms. This patient could also read normally, and he could spell nonwords and very regular words correctly, but was flummoxed by even very common irregular words. G.R. had a well-developed phonological spelling strategy, but his orthographic spelling strategy didn't work. These two cases show that the phonological and the orthographic spelling strategies can function independently of each other.

These cases give us interesting insight into the normal spelling process, but we can't really generalize from them to children suffering from dyslexia. In cases of agraphia we have to do with a person, generally an adult, who has learned to read and write normally but who is unable to do so today. In cases of dyslexia we have to do with reading and writing systems that have never been fully developed. As with word-decoding, we feel spelling is in the main performed by using either the phonological or the orthographic strategy (Frith, 1980). Yet we are aware that most dyslexics cannot be categorized unambiguously as one or the other on the basis of the types of spelling errors they commit (Seymour and Porpodas, 1980).

Spelling strategies and linguistic aspects of words

Words come in different types, and there are certain linguistic aspects of words that account for how well a given strategy will yield the correct spelling. These aspects include such factors as whether the word is long or short, regular or irregularly spelled, and whether the word occurs very frequently in the texts the reader has been working with, or whether it is a word of low frequency.

When the speller tries to spell a word by using *the orthographic strategy*, we find these effects on the various types of words:

1. Regular and irregular words are spelled equally well.
2. Highly frequent words are correctly spelled much more often than the uncommon words.
3. There is a very large word/nonword discrepancy; that is, real words are much more often spelled correctly than nonwords.
4. Word-length has little effect. There is no appreciable difference in the percentage of correct spellings for short words than for long words.

When the speller uses *the phonological strategy*, we find this pattern of errors:

1. Irregular words are much more prone to be spelled wrong, and we see examples of the pupil regularizing irregular words, e.g. spelling *photo*   as *foto*, or *ball* as *bal*.
2. No clear effect of word-frequency; i.e. highly frequent words are not spelled any better than very uncommon words.
3. No clear word/nonword discrepancy effect; i.e., words and nonwords are spelled equally well.
4. Length has an effect. Long words are more often misspelled than short words.

Determining which types of words the pupil has the most trouble with can tell us about the strategy he or she is using.

Auxiliary strategies

The two main spelling strategies are sometimes inadequate. There are several other strategies spellers use for extra help in trying to figure out a word:

Finding analogies. Knowing how *boat* and *coat* are spelled, the pupil who is trying to write *moat* may well hit upon the solution by thinking of these analogous rhyming words.

Visual-orthographic recognition. Writing the word on scratch paper to see if it looks right.

Morphemic analysis. Looking to see if the word, or parts of it, are grammatical transformations of morphemes that the speller knows how to spell. For example, if the speller wants to write *national*, he or she might notice that it 'comes from' *nation*, even though the pronunciation is different.

Verbal memorizing. Sometimes the sound of the word being spelled is particularly memorable. The distinctive cadence in the sound of the letters in *Mississippi* being read off has helped many a student get the spelling right. Some people remember spellings by remembering 'wrong' pronunciations: *to+get+her* for *together* or *pe+ople* for *people*

Motoric memory. Sometimes hands can remember things minds forget. A word can have a strong kinesthetic identity for a pupil, and he or she can write it better without thinking about the spelling.

Guessing. One of the talents skilled spellers have, is that they can make good, educated guesses.

Spellers often choose more than one strategy when attacking a hard word. When trying to spell the word *bespeckled*, the writer might take this mixed line of reasoning: The first syllable is probably spelled *be-*, this being a fairly common morpheme denoting something like 'marked by', and well known in words like *bewail, bemoan, bewitched* and *bewildered.* (This is a mix of morphemic and analogy strategies, and it succeeds in ruling out other ways of representing the first syllable, such as *bea* or *bie*.) The root of the word is *speckle*; that being a fairly well-known word, although it is most common in its plural form, *speckles*. (The orthographic strategy, using a morphemic line of reasoning to get rid of the *s*.) And the suffix is *-d*, the usual way of rendering the past participle morpheme, which here will indicate the desired adjectival meaning. (Again, the morphemic strategy, with a morphosyntactical twist.)

Throughout the whole process the speller has probably been using the phonological strategy to zero in on the morphemes: Hearing the word *bespeckled* in the mind's ear, the writer knew it would start with a *b-*, this letter being just about the only way of rendering the initial sound /b/; perhaps this insight led to the morphemic insight that yielded *be-*, or perhaps the reader found the *be-* morpheme first, and used the phonological strategy to double-check. The same thing would have happened with the start of the root, *sp-*, and perhaps the root's first vowel, *-e-* : phonological thinking alone could yield them, even though it couldn't yield the whole word. Being able to use two strategies to generate some of the graphemes makes the spelling process much more successful. And sometimes we see a third strategy used to check the whole word: the speller jots the word down, looks at it, finds that it looks familiar (the visual-orthographic strategy, a variation on the orthographic strategy).

The degree to which pupils learn to use these strategies depends on how much emphasis the teacher puts on correct spellings and the strategies for achieving them. It is important that the teacher understands how spelling skills develop, so that the child's normal misspellings at one stage are not interpreted as a sign of any special spelling difficulty.

A Model of the Spelling Process

As with word-decoding, it is possible to analyze closely how the various subprocesses in spelling fit together, and to present this conception of the complete spelling process in a model. Figure 3.1 shows the main features of our conception of spelling. It is based on the traditional dual-route thinking, but it specifies more precisely than usual the separate subprocesses involved in the spelling strategies.

The orthographic spelling strategy is indicated by the bold arrows, while the phonological route is represented by the light-faced arrows. The circles represent the various mental subprocesses that take place during the use of these two strategies.

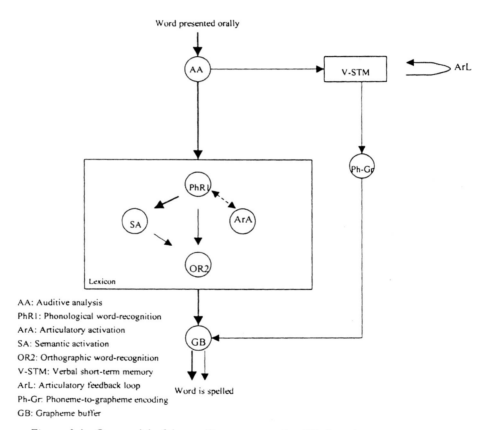

AA: Auditive analysis
PhRI: Phonological word-recognition
ArA: Articulatory activation
SA: Semantic activation
OR2: Orthographic word-recognition
V-STM: Verbal short-term memory
ArL: Articulatory feedback loop
Ph-Gr: Phoneme-to-grapheme encoding
GB: Grapheme buffer

Figure 3.1. Our model of the spelling process, simplified version.
Bold-faced arrows indicate the orthographic strategy, light arrows the
phonological.

Spelling of a dictated word with a familiar spelling

Let us say that the pupil is asked to write down a word the teacher has dictated. If the pupil knows how the word is spelled, then he or she can take the orthographic route. Figure 3.2 illustrates the processes involved.

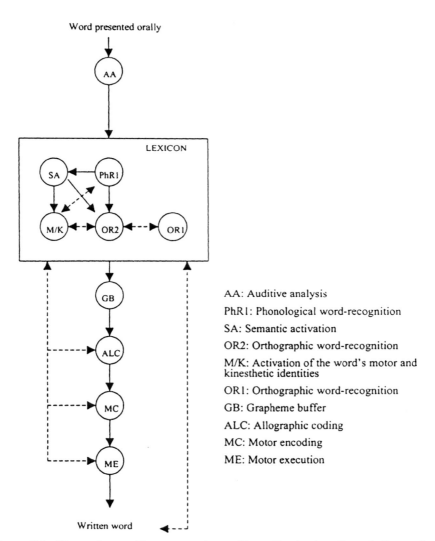

AA: Auditive analysis

PhR1: Phonological word-recognition

SA: Semantic activation

OR2: Orthographic word-recognition

M/K: Activation of the word's motor and kinesthetic identities

OR1: Orthographic word-recognition

GB: Grapheme buffer

ALC: Allographic coding

MC: Motor encoding

ME: Motor execution

Figure 3.2. The orthographic strategy in spelling. The broken lines indicate the associations between subprocesses and the influence of feedback from the cognitive system.

The child hears the word that the teacher reads aloud, and performs an auditive analysis (AA) of the sounds. The sounds are recognized as a word the child knows (PhR1). These first two subprocesses are linguistic skills the child has acquired years before beginning school. The child's phonological recognition of the word then triggers the activation of the word's orthographic identity (OR2); that is, the child recalls or retrieves the spelling of the written word. At the same time, the word's semantic identity is activated (SA). In the case of homophonic words, e.g. *right* and *write*, both orthographic identities are activated, and both semantic identities as well. Here, the child uses the grammatical or semantic context to decide between the two. (To keep the model as simple as possible, we have not included a grammatical component.)

The activation of the word's orthographic identity then causes the graphemes in the spelling of the word to be brought into consciousness and be stored in the grapheme buffer (GB), the location of the short-term memory for graphemes. In order to write the graphemes, their motor identities are activated (MC). These motor identities are bits of stored knowledge in the lexicon; they contain a precise set of instructions for the motions needed to form the letters. Finally, the sequence of movements is executed (ME). The word is written.

For the sake of clarity, we have treated the subprocesses individually and sequentially. In reality, however, they interact, and the job done by a particular subprocess is determined not only by its input from the subprocess before it, but by continuous feedback from the cognitive system.

We should also note the importance of the word's motor-kinesthetic and visual identities. The word's motor-kinesthetic identity - how the word feels when you write it - can let the speller's hand just write the word, almost by itself. And while the word is being written, the speller's recollection of the word's visual identity is used to check the spelling, to see if the word just written looks familiar or if something has gone wrong. In Figure 3.2, this is shown by the feedback arrows running from the two motor processes MC and ME to the motor-kinesthetic identity in the lexicon, and by the feedback arrow between the spelled word and the word's orthographic identity (OR1).

Spelling of a dictated word with an unfamiliar spelling

If the pupil does not know how a word is spelled, he or she cannot use the orthographic strategy. Then the phonological strategy is necessary. Figure 3.3 shows the subprocesses that make up the phonological route.

The first two subprocesses, the auditive analysis (AA) and the phonological word-recognition (PhR1), are the same as in the orthographic strategy.

The activation of the word's phonological identity in PhR1 gives the writer access to the word's semantic identity (SA), but because the writer has not yet learned how to spell this word, there is no sequence of graphemes in OR2 to be retrieved. The function fails. (This is represented in the model by the shading on OR2.)

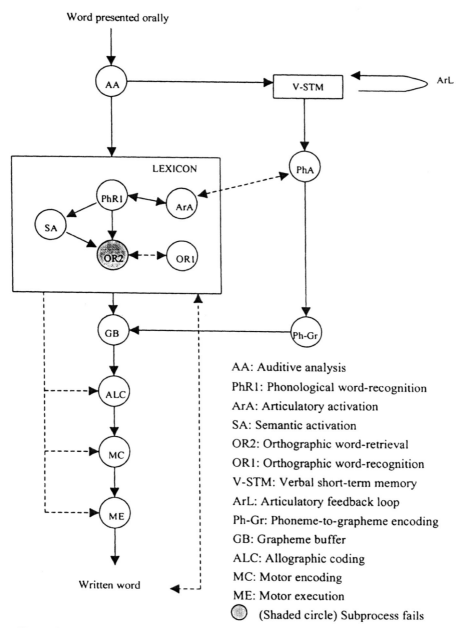

Figure 3.3. The phonological strategy used when spelling a regular word when the spelling is unfamiliar to the writer.

Pretty much in tandem with this unsuccessful process, a back-up process has started, one that will lead to the unfamiliar word being correctly spelled.

The auditive analysis is not only outputted to the PhR1, it is also outputted to the verbal short-term memory (VSTM), where it is both stored and outputted to phonological analysis (PhA). Here the word is broken down into smaller units, phonemes and (perhaps) highly frequent consonant-clusters (*tr, br*, etc.). The verbal short-term memory is actually a complicated subprocess, full of numerous sub-subproceses. Here the sounds, as yet not broken down into units, are stored. The articulatory loop (ArL) we have drawn at the VSTM is meant to indicate that we often need to say the word aloud or to ourselves in order to remember the sounds it contains while the phonological analysis is taking place; it often seems that the short-term memory needs to be refreshed every moment or two to keep the sounds in the right order. (In reality this process is more complicated than we have indicated. Some sort of a phoneme buffer is involved, but we have chosen not to illustrate this for fear of cluttering up the model.)

The phoneme analysis (PhA) makes use of not only phonological information, but articulatory information as well. Parallel to the activation of the word's phonological identity at PhR1, the articulatory identity of the word is activated at ArA. The articulatory information is crucial for a correct phonological analysis, especially of the consonants. The phoneme-to-grapheme recoding process (Ph-Gr) selects the appropriate graphemes. A deficient short-term memory will hinder this recoding greatly, thereby weakening the entire phonological route. Moreover, the recoding into graphemes can be helped by lexical processes. If the child is asked e.g. to spell *national*, he or she may recognize the root-morpheme *nation*, and start from there.

The activated graphemes are stored a moment or two in the grapheme buffer (GB) while the motor encoding takes place (MC). Finally, the movements are carried out (ME); the word is written.

Spelling of dictated nonwords

The phonological strategy is used when we are confronted with words we do not know how to spell. Nonwords, which by definition we have never seen nor heard before, fall into the same category. The process of spelling nonwords is much the same as for real words that the writer recognizes, but does not know how to spell. But there are some differences. Figure 3.4 shows the subprocesses involved when we attempt to write nonwords.

The dictated nonword is again analyzed, but when the result is outputted to phonological word-recognition (PhR) the system draws a blank. No recognition takes place, so no semantic activation (SA) can happen; the spelling can neither be recalled (OR2) nor is there any spelling to recognize (OR1).

The sound-input is stored in the verbal short-term memory (VSTM), where, again, the articulation loop (ArL) helps keep the mental image of the sound of the word intact while the phonological analysis (PhA) is going on. The repeated articulation (done either physically or mentally) of the nonword is important not only for the *input* to the phonological analysis; it seems to provide *direct support* for the analysis as well. Comparing Figures 3.4 and 3.3 we see the difference between real words and nonwords: in 3.3 the real word's sound-identity, its articulation, and

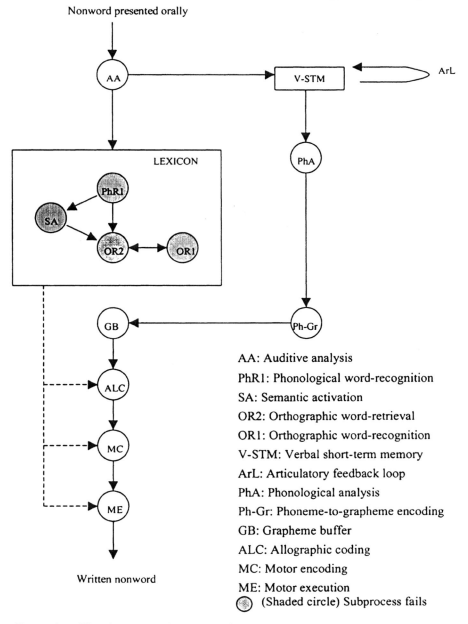

AA: Auditive analysis
PhR1: Phonological word-recognition
SA: Semantic activation
OR2: Orthographic word-retrieval
OR1: Orthographic word-recognition
V-STM: Verbal short-term memory
ArL: Articulatory feedback loop
PhA: Phonological analysis
Ph-Gr: Phoneme-to-grapheme encoding
GB: Grapheme buffer
ALC: Allographic coding
MC: Motor encoding
ME: Motor execution
(Shaded circle) Subprocess fails

Figure 3.4. The phonological strategy when attempting to spell nonwords.

its meaning were all active, and these activations could provide support to the phonological analysis. It is easier to analyze the sounds in a word you've heard before and know what means than it is to pick out the phonemes in an unfamiliar string of word-like sounds. This is probably the reason that even good spellers have the feeling of having to 'think twice' when proposing spellings of nonwords, and why they might have to consciously repeat the nonword several times while figuring out a probable spelling for it. With no semantic ideas as a hook to 'hang' the nonword on, all you have to go on is its pronunciation.

Being able to break the sound of a word or nonword down into its constituent phonemes is essential for the use of the phonological strategy. A deficit in phoneme-analysis will be seen as a lot of misspellings of nonwords and real words that are of low frequency in the types of texts the person has been reading.

The phoneme-to-grapheme recoding process is also essential. Here we have to remember the essential lack of symmetry between spelling and reading. The reader, working from the graphemes, only has to get the sound right (or nearly right) to trigger a recognition of the word. A good reader confronted for the first time with the word *mite* shouldn't have any problem reading it off as /majt/, even if he hasn't seen this word before. There are literally hundreds of words with the spelling-pattern consonant - *i* - consonant - *e*, so the 'long *i*' sound should pop up pretty quickly. But working the other way around, from the sound /majt/ to graphemes that can represent it, the writer has several possible spellings to choose from: *might*, or *mite*, even (depending on the speller's accent), *mate*, *mait* or *maite*. Being aware of how sounds can be encoded in graphemes, and knowing that there often is more than one way to do it, is called *graphemic awareness*, a type of knowledge many poor spellers lack.

To write the word, the mental idea of the graphemes has to be recoded into motor processes. A deficiency in the motor system can lead to a poorly formed word. Poorly functioning fine motor skills or weak eye-to-hand coordination are common culprits. Nonetheless, we need to remember that the illegible handwriting we often see in children is more often due to more prosaic deficiencies, such as lack of practice, or an embedded desire to camouflage uncertain spellings or flee the building. Emotional blocks can also hinder good penmanship, something that often shows itself in uneven pressure on the pencil and wildly uneven size of letters. For dyslexics, the act of writing is so fraught with bad feelings that we shouldn't be surprised when this is abundantly apparent in their handwriting.

Writing non-dictated words

When the pupil wants to write a word that hasn't been dictated, the situation is somewhat different. It is shown in Figure 3.5. Here, the spelling process starts with an activation in the lexicon (SA). The pupil wants to present a thought on paper, and he or she searches for the string of phonemes, i.e. the word, that can best express this thought. When the right phonological identity is activated, the writer can decide which route to take, the phonological (if he or she doesn't know the spelling) or the orthographic (if the spelling is known).

The Writing Process

Writing well is not just a question of spelling well. Writing well entails getting one's thoughts down on paper in an organized, understandable and cogent way, and this is a much more complicated process than mere spelling. Because the problems dyslexic children have are not confined to spelling and handwriting, we need to say something about these more complex processes.

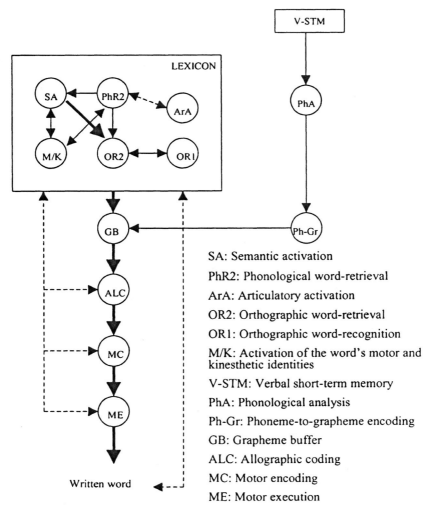

SA: Semantic activation

PhR2: Phonological word-retrieval

ArA: Articulatory activation

OR2: Orthographic word-retrieval

OR1: Orthographic word-recognition

M/K: Activation of the word's motor and kinesthetic identities

V-STM: Verbal short-term memory

PhA: Phonological analysis

Ph-Gr: Phoneme-to-grapheme encoding

GB: Grapheme buffer

ALC: Allographic coding

MC: Motor encoding

ME: Motor execution

Figure 3.5. Strategies when spelling a non-dictated word.
The orthographic strategy is indicated by bold-faced lines, while the phonological route is indicated by lighter lines.

The most influential cognitive model of the writing process is the model formulated by Hayes and Fowler (1980). Their model is based on an analysis of what adult writers say when they think out loud while writing. (This is called the 'Thinking out loud' protocol.) Hayes and Fowler identified three main components of the writing process: Planning, execution, and revision. These components do not always occur in that order; they all occur many times throughout the writing process. For example, while writing (executing) a passage, the writer might be consciously planning the next passage, while at the same time looking back in the text to make revisions of earlier passages. So the planning component is not necessarily finished before the writing itself starts, and the revision isn't necessarily started after the whole piece is written down.

This model is most applicable for advanced writing. In order to adapt it to the neophyte's or the dyslexic's painstaking efforts at composition, the model will have to be adjusted. Berninger (1996) has attempted this, with interesting results.

The execution phase pointed out by Hayes and Fowler can be divided into two parts: text generation and text transcription. Text generation is the phase where thoughts and ideas acquire linguistic form and get stored in the working memory. The transcription is the writing down part; the thoughts are transcribed, as it were. In some children we see an apparent discrepancy between these two phases: some children have a lot they want to write, but perhaps because they have so much on their minds, what they actually get down on paper is incoherent and fragmentary.

With regard to the planning phase, Berninger finds it fruitful to posit two types of planning for young writers, the advanced pre-planning of whole paragraphs and the on-going, immediate 'on-line' planning that takes place concurrently with the writing. Similarly, the revision can take place during the writing, or afterward, when the whole paragraph can be checked.

When children start to learn to write, they do not plan very far ahead. Typically, their planning is the on-line type. They wait until they have written one sentence before thinking up the next one. Pupils who are having a hard time getting the hang of writing do not typically revise much, neither while they are writing a passage nor afterward. Children generally become authors before they become editors.

Writing makes demands on the pupil's long-term memory, for it is from memory that the child finds the thoughts and ideas to be expressed in writing. Here are stored the bits of knowledge about the world, the *semantic memory*, and the *episodic memory*, which is responsible for remembering the personal stories that make up one's sense of one's self. Here too is the *procedural memory*, which stores the 'how to' instructions needed for, among other things, writing; and the *perceptual representation memory*, which stores the mental images of letters and words. At least equally important is the short-term *working memory*, which gains in importance as the young writer matures. A writer who cannot keep relevant thoughts in orderly bundles is a writer who will easily lose his or her train of thought; then inchoate ideas get scattered to the winds and communication breaks down.

Another decisive hindrance to the young writer is a lack of *automaticity* in the various subprocesses that constitute writing. If the physical act of writing is too tedious due to uncertain motor-skills, or the spellings of the common words that make up most of any text are too elusive, then the composition will probably suffer. If these sorts of subprocesses have to be closely attended to, then too little mental capacity will be left for finding and ordering the ideas the child wants to express.

With regard to reading, we have already underlined the importance of practice, which is the only way to gain the automaticity that is the hallmark of the good reader. The only way to become a good reader is to read a lot, and the only way to become a good writer is through writing a lot. Practice may not make perfect, but it surely makes better. The pity is that those who need to practice the most - dyslexic children - are the very ones who do so the least. With their ugly handwriting and bizarre spellings, they feel that they seldom manage to write anything worth reading; indeed, some children are not even able read what they themselves have written. Given these conditions, the usefulness of writing as a means of communication approaches zero. When even short post-it notes and diary entries are threatening endeavors, then writing book reports, stories, and pen-pal letters is impossible. Confronted with tasks like these, it is easy to throw in the towel.

Yet giving up writing is in some respects tantamount to giving up thinking. It is therefore essential that we understand that the writing problems of dyslexic children are much more serious than their ugly handwriting and bizarre spellings. When working with dyslexics we need to devote more time and effort to writing. We return to this subject when treating teaching methods in Chapter 8.

Brief Summary

We can look at spelling from two perspectives. First of all, we can look at it as a socially necessary skill in our literate culture. Secondly, we can look at spelling as a window into the child's mental lexicon and his or her use of the various strategies of spelling. In this chapter we have concentrated on the latter perspective. We have looked at the stages spellers go through, and tried to characterize each of the stages. This developmental model also included a system of error analysis based on four types of words. We have also discussed various types of spelling errors, and examined them in light of the pupils' speech habits. We have seen that dyslexics do not have qualitatively different misspellings than normal pupils, they just have more of them. But dyslexics do have bad handwriting.

We assume, on good evidence, that there are two main strategies for spelling a word, the orthographic and the phonological strategy. In order to use the orthographic strategy, the writer has to have the spelling stored in his or her mental lexicon. This enables the spelling to be retrieved when needed. This strategy allows both regular and irregular words to be spelled correctly.

When using the phonological strategy, the sound of the word is first analyzed (phonemic segmenting), then recoded into graphemes. This strategy allows the writer to spell words he or she hasn't yet learned how to spell, as long as the words' spellings are fairly regular.

Based on these two strategies, we have presented a series of models which show how the various types of words can be spelled. Models such as these can

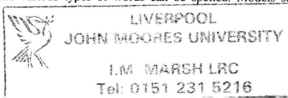

provide us with a theoretical foundation for developing diagnostic methods.

We have also looked at the more complicated dimensions of the entire writing process, and we have pointed out how the dyslexic child's general problems with writing arise in part as a result of problems with spelling and handwriting, and are in part due to problems with working memory and concentration. These problems in turn have a negative impact on the young writer's ability to plan, execute, and revise written work.

CHAPTER 4

DYSLEXIA AND PHONOLOGY

We have pointed out many times in this book that dyslexia is the result of a linguistic problem, and that phonological skills are of great importance in learning to read and write. Individuals with dyslexia usually have a disturbance in the phonological system, and this disturbance is manifested by:

> problems in segmenting words into phonemes
> problems in keeping linguistic material (strings of sounds or letters) in the short-term memory
> problems in repeating back long nonwords
> problems in reading and writing even short nonwords
> problems in naming colours, numbers, and things in pictures quickly
> a slower rate of speech, sometimes with an indistinct pronunciation
> problems in playing word-games where the point is to manipulate phonemes (games like Pig-Latin: *Ankay ooya eekspay Igpay Atinlay?* Or spoonerisms, such as Inspector Clouseau's *A writ of fellous jadge* for *A fit of jealous rage*).

Strangely enough, this phonological deficit is very limited in scope; people can have a marked deficiency in dealing with phonemes yet still have perfectly good cognitive abilities in all other areas (Moats, 1996). Even their other linguistic functions can be quite normal, or even better than average. Dyslexics can live normal lives despite their handicap, and some few of them even manage to do well in school and at university. Their deficit can perhaps best be conceived of as a reduced function in a special module in the cognitive-linguistic system. This module, which we appear to be born with, is responsible for dealing with the sound-system of the spoken language. Under normal linguistic conditions, when the person is speaking or listening to others, the phonological deficit is not noticeable. But when conditions demand a higher degree of function in the processing of sounds, for example when speaking Pig-Latin, reciting back long nonwords, or trying to decipher Inspector Clouseau, then the problem rears its ugly head. The demands made on the phonological module when performing these activities are very much the same as when learning to read and write.

In this chapter we will be looking at these disturbances in the phonological system and we will see how important phonology is for development of reading skills. We will see how early signs of phonological problems in preschool can be omens of coming reading problems in first or second grade and later. And we will also be looking at whether it is possible or feasible to prevent reading and writing problems in the early grades by taking measures already in preschool.

Why is reading and writing so difficult for some children to deal with? In order to understand what is going on when a child fails to learn to deal with written language, we need to look closely at the specific cognitive and linguistic demands that writing makes, demands that are different from those *speaking* makes. Let us start by making some general comparisons between writing and speech.

All societies ever discovered have a fully developed oral language, but only comparatively few societies have systems of writing. In these comparatively few 'literate' societies we find that there always are some individuals who master speaking and listening, but cannot master reading and writing.

In the history of human development, just as in the child's development, oral language comes first. Only later does written language appear. Oral language is a part of our biological baggage. Writing, on the other hand, is an intensely cultural product, and it only appeared some few thousands of years ago.

All natural, human languages function in very much the same way: a finite number of vowel-sounds and consonant-sounds, usually two to four dozen, are combined in various systematic ways.

In order to learn to talk, the only thing a child has to do is be around people who talk. But in order to learn to read, the child almost always has to submit to some kind of 'teaching' - in school, or less formally by a parent or an older sibling.

We see, then, that writing and speech are not truly analogous functions. Learning to talk is as natural as learning to walk or learning to experience depth perception. Learning to read is more like learning to play chess or program a computer.

In addition to being able to speak and understand the speech of others, what other talents does a child need to learn to read? To understand this problem we will need to look more closely at the nature of language. Consonants and vowels are the basic building-blocks, the phonological components, of a child's natural language-acts. Contrary to popular opinion, phonemes must not be thought of as the sounds themselves. Phonemes are the abstract 'categories' we sort the sounds of utterances into, the control units we use when we produce and perceive speech. For the natural user of spoken language, these categories exist only on a subconscious level. As we know, you do not have to consciously know anything at all about phonemes in order to carry on a conversation.

Phonemes help convey meaning, yet are meaningless in themselves. The three phonemes in the word *dog*, for instance, do not have anything 'doglike' about them, either individually or in combination. But if you change one of them, for instance by substituting the *d* for a *b*, you get a different word, in this case *bog*, or you get a phoneme-string with no conventional meaning. This, incidentally, is how the set of phonemes of a language is defined. We know that /b/ and /d/ are different phonemes in English because we find pairs of words where the only difference in sound is that one member of the pair has a /b/ where the other member has a /d/, *bog* and *dog*, or *bobby* and *body*. Or to take a more subtle example: voiced and unvoiced *s*, /z/ and /s/, are two different phonemes in English because there exist pairs of words (in English) which are pronounced exactly the same, except for the difference in voicing of the *s*-sounds. Examples of such *minimal pairs*, as these words are called, would be *hiss* (pronounced /his/) and *his* (/hiz/), or *miss* (/mis/) and *Ms.* (/miz/). Because the difference in voicing of the two *s*-sounds is semantically significant, linguists agree that they are two different phonemes.

But the situation is a bit more confusing, because not all sound differences are semantically significant. In the previous chapter, in connection with the dog named *SBOT*, we noted the difference between aspirated and unaspirated /p/. In some positions, for instance immediately after an /s/, the little puff of air we usually emit at the end of the /p/ is subpressed, as in the word *spill* or *Spot*. This phonological difference is not used in the English sound system to separate between different words, so it does not warrant cleaving *p*'s into two different phonemes. (Linguists call the difference in aspiration of the phoneme /p/ a non-functional, sub-phonemic positional variation, and the two versions of /p/ are called *allophones.*)

Phonemes, then, are what we use to create meaning. Even young children, who have no concept of what a phoneme is, have an implicit wealth of knowledge about the phonemes of their language. If they didn't, they wouldn't understand speech.

There are around 40 phonemes in English, give or take a few depending on which dialect we are looking at. Estimates of the number of words in the English language generally number in excess of 400,000. The function of phonology is to form these 400,000 words by combining the 40 or so small, meaningless and abstract phonemes into one or the other of the 400,000 words. Phonemes by themselves may not mean anything, but when they are put in the right order they can mean just about anything under the sun.

Conveying meaning through the combination of discrete units is a marvelous invention, and it is very unlike the conventional systems of signals we find in other species, for example the dancing of honeybees upon returning to the hive. In these primitive signaling systems, each item of information is represented by a unique, conventional gesture. Imagine what a human language would be like if each word consisted of just one unique sound. It would probably be impossible for such a language to develop a vocabulary numbering more than a few hundred words.

When children begin to learn to read, they have to be able to deal with phonology more consciously than when they learned to speak. They need to understand the alphabetical principle, that is, to understand that the phonemes of a word can be represented by letters, and that the differences between words is heard in the phonological structures that the letters of written words encode.

Why is it so difficult for some children to understand this principle, and to gain conscious access to the phonology they already master so well in their spoken language?

Here we need to take yet another step into the world of phonetics, and look at how speakers produce phonemes and how listeners hear them. We generally analyze the sounds of words sequentially, one phoneme after the other, as in /spil/ or

/hiz/, as indeed we write words sequentially with letters, *spill* or *his*. But spoken language is, as we mentioned previously, marked by a high degree of *co-articulation*.

Phonemes, when we produce them, are movements in the organs of speech. For example, a /b/ is a closing and opening of the lips, accompanied by an explosion of breath and voicing. But before we are finished with one phoneme, our speech organs have usually begun preparing for the next phoneme. If you are going to say *book*, you close your lips with a slight rounding, because you 'know' your next phoneme is a vowel-sound that needs rounded lips. If you are going to say *beetle*, you don't close your lips rounded, but laterally spread, in anticipation of the bright *ee*-sound. And so it goes all through the utterance, with sounds blurring, overlapping and interfering with each other. So when we represent words with sequentially written letters, we are really only telling half the story (McGuiness, 1997).

Why is spoken language so complex? Surely it would have been easier for listeners if all the speakers pronounced their utterances as strings of discrete, tidy, unblurred phonemes. Here we should again remember that speech has been around much longer than print, and that speech is obviously the result of a long biological evolution. The good thing about co-articulation is that it lets us speak much faster than if we carefully articulated words one phoneme at a time, and this speed seems to have given us a biological advantage. We usually speak at the rate of 10 to 20 phonemes per second - much, much faster than if we delivered phonemes one at a time, like pearls on a string.

Another advantage of co-articulation is that it provides a higher degree of redundancy. The vowel-sound in *book* is incorporated in both of the surrounding consonant-sounds, so if the listener doesn't hear the vowel, e.g. because of some extraneous noise, then nothing is lost. The listener still hears the word *book*. So the redundancy that is created by co-articulation helps guard against what communication engineers call *noise* - the inevitable background buzz that accompanies any signal.

Just like other specialized cognitive processes that have evolved over great spans of time (another example is depth perception), co-articulation is fully automatic. Neither speakers nor listeners have to know anything at all about it, we just do it. Speakers need only to think of what they are saying, and listeners to what is being said. Phonemes get chosen, blended, and spoken; then heard, unblended, and understood automatically. By way of a preliminary conclusion we can say that our specialized phonological module takes care of these tasks for us.

Normally there is nothing in children's natural experience with spoken language that would lead them to discover the alphabetic principle by themselves. An emergent reader has no spontaneous reason to discover that the word *book* contains three different phonemes. Children normally hear words as acoustic bundles where the *meaning* is the point, and the *sounds*, as it were, are transparent. In conversation, you are *supposed to* see through the sounds to get at the import of what the person is saying.

Nor is it possible to pick out the phonemes merely by listening; co-articulation makes this difficult. Saying 'buh ooo kuh' doesn't help either, because that just doesn't sound like *book*. Gaining access to the level of phonemes is never a question of 'just listening'. It is a question of gradually understanding, discovering, and becoming aware of the intricate interplay of meaning with sounds. While most people achieve this insight without problem, some individuals, despite massive help, just don't 'get it'. It appears that this defect is sharply limited in scope, because some children with fine talents in other areas can only achieve a modest measure of phonological awareness with great difficulty.

We will now turn to some studies that have shown how a lack of phonemic awareness and reading problems are associated.

If it is the case that learning to read makes specific demands on the child's phonological system, is it then possible to predict early on which children will have trouble learning to read and write when they start school? An early diagnosis of children at risk would make it possible to start remedial measures even before they start to fail at school.

Can Reading and Writing Problems be Predicted in Preschoolers?

Scarborough (1990) studied 32 children of dyslexic parents. She followed the children's development from age 2 1/2 to 8 years. As many as 65 percent were diagnosed as dyslexic at age 8, which indicates that the disorder has a strong genetic component. Already at 2 1/2 years they evinced measurable linguistic disturbances. Their grammar skills and pronunciation were less well developed than a control group of children with normal-reading parents. By age 3 1/2 they had a poorer understanding of words and a poorer ability to come up with the names of items on picture-cards than their cohorts had. And by age 5 they knew fewer of the letters of the alphabet, had less phonological awareness, and knew the names of fewer items than the controls.

Scarborough's study shows that there are early warning signs in the child's linguistic development that signal impending reading and writing problems at school.

Other researchers have also studied children of dyslexic parents. Locke's study (Locke, 1997) is not finished yet, so we don't know how many of his study group will wind up dyslexic. But the preliminary results are interesting. Locke started studying the children when they were 8 *months* old. He registered and phonetically analyzed their babbling. Strangely, even at this early age there were differences in how at-risk children and a control group (with normal-reading parents) dealt with language-sounds. The at-risk children babbled with fewer different sounds and less complex sequences of sounds. Locke's hypothesis is that children with a strong genetic disposition for dyslexia show a different linguistic development: they base more of their understanding on social signals and contextual information, and derive less information from segmenting and manipulating phonetic segments.

Snowling has also studied very young at-risk children (Snowling and Nation, 1977). She submitted 71 preschoolers (with dyslexic parents) to comprehensive language tests. The children were 3 1/2 years old. Snowling found, as did Scarborough, that at-risk children had more difficulty repeating back nonwords than children in the control group. She showed the children pictures of imaginary animals which she gave fanciful, nonword names to. The at-risk children were less adept at using these names, and they had less knowledge of letters and knew fewer rhymes and jingles than the controls.

Elbro, Petersen, and Borström (1988) have also employed the strategy of studying children of dyslexic parents. They followed 49 at-risk children from the start of kindergarten (age 6) to the start of second grade (age 8), at which time it is possible to diagnose dyslexia.

In accordance with the other studies, they found that the children whose parents had reading problems had a much greater chance of developing dyslexia than children with normal-reading parents, and that the level of linguistic competency at kindergarten age is a clear predictor of dyslexia. In particular, they found that children's skills with the sounds of language predict later reading problems. In addition to making various measurements of the children's phonological and morphological awareness, they designed a clever experiment to measure how distinct the children's mental representations of the sounds of words were. They did this by getting the children to interact with a hand-puppet who spoke with a speech impediment, and asking the children to teach the puppet how to pronounce the words correctly.

Among all the tasks they used to chart the linguistic prowess of their kindergarten group, Elbro and his co-workers found that the important skills for learning to read and write were: letter knowledge, phoneme identification, phoneme subtraction, verbal short-term memory, having well-defined mental representations of the sounds of words, being able to pronounce difficult words precisely, and having a capacious passive vocabulary. All of these were important, but one factor stood out as clearly the most important of all: having distinct mental representations of the sounds of words. When all other variables were controlled, this one factor alone could account for much of the child's success or failure at learning to read.

Lundberg, Olofsson and Wall (1980) showed that it is possible to predict with a high degree of certainty at preschool age how a children will fare in reading instruction when they start school. Among all the various tests they used, it was their test of phonological awareness that was the best predictor. Many subsequent studies have confirmed these findings (e.g. Badian, 1994; Blachman, 1984; Bradley and Bryant, 1985; Hurford et al., 1994; Torgesen, Morgan and Davis, 1992).

To sum up, we can say that children who are genetically disposed to becoming dyslexics show a delay or a deficit primarily in their phonological development. Their internal representations of what words sound like are fuzzy and lacking in detail (Brady, 1997). Moreover, it is not easy for them to move their attention from the meaning of a word to its form: to what it sounds like, and how it is constructed. These phonological problems make learning to read and write an exceptionally difficult task (cf. Rack et al., 1994).

The Problem of Identifying At-risk Children

When research has so unequivocally shown the strong connection between phonological development and later reading and writing ability, then why don't we instigate massive screening programmes, so that we can put all the soon-to-be-dyslexic preschoolers into a remedial programme. That way we can cure the problem before it becomes a problem.

This may sound like a good idea, but on reflection it is not that easy. It is true that research has shown a strong association between poor phonological abilities during preschool and later problems with writing. In fact, the correlation found in the studies is generally around 0.80. Statistically that is considered a 'good correlation'. But here we have to be clear about the difference between making good predictions about a group and forming good prognoses for individuals.

We can look at it this way: Suppose that we give a test-battery to 1000 preschoolers. 100 of them score so poorly that we predict that they will develop dyslexia. A year later, when they are in school, we find that 80 of the 100 are in fact dyslexic; our prediction was impressively accurate. Of the 900 children who tested normal, we find that 800 are indeed reading normally; again, our prediction turned out to be pretty accurate. As group-level predictions, these are good. But we need to look at it from another perspective. 20 of the children we predicted would be dyslexic turned out to be normal readers, and 100 of the children we thought would learn to read normally, have instead turned out to be dyslexic. So of the 180 children who actually developed reading problems, we discovered only 80 in our preschool screening. That is less than half. Table 4.1 presents this graphically:

Table 4.1. Accuracy in classifying preschoolers as at-risk students.

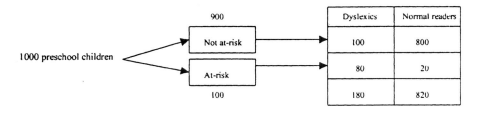

	Dyslexics	Normal readers
900		
Not at-risk	100	800
1000 preschool children	80	20
At-risk		
100	180	820

Another question the notion of preschool screenings raises is the dilemma of 'false positives'. There were 20 children who we predicted would develop dyslexia, but who turned out to read normally. Will labeling them as 'probable dyslexics' be detrimental them?

The idea of an early identification and remediation of reading problems exerts a powerful emotional tug on all of us. Yet there are two conditions that would have to be fulfilled before any sort of screening programme should be implemented. First of all, we have to be fairly certain that we can do something constructive with the probable dyslexics. Secondly, we need to be sure that no great ill will befall our false positives.

Given the state of our knowledge and capability today, we advise caution. The inadequacy of our individual prognoses can have many causes. Any sort of testing of preschool children is always a bit chancy: Some children are inattentive, others lack stamina, while others may not have been listening when the instructions were given. Or the test itself may not be statistically reliable. But above all, we just do not know enough about the causes of dyslexia to be able to devise really good diagnostic tools. In addition, we know that preschool children develop at different rates. Some of the ones who are lagging behind in phonological skills when we test them in preschool may develop enough of these skills before they start school to be able to profit from reading instruction.

A Longitudinal Study

In a Danish study, nearly 400 children were followed from preschool to fourth grade (Lundberg, Frost and Petersen, 1988). They were tested for various skills at regular intervals throughout the nearly five years of the study. At the end of third grade a study group of 35 dyslexic pupils (25 boys and 10 girls) was selected on the basis of their low scores on a comprehensive battery of tests. These tests required them to read silently words and sentences, and to spell words. In addition, they were given a standard intelligence test (Raven).

The researchers wanted to know how these dyslexic students had developed since preschool, compared to the rest of the children who were reading normally. Do dyslexic students have a different kind of linguistic development than the others? Among the tests that were given at regular intervals to the total group of 400 were tests of phonological awareness. These included tasks such as deleting the first phoneme in a word, counting the number of phonemes in words, and blending a string of phonemes to make a word. These tests were given three times, in September and May of their last year before starting school, and in September of first grade. The results for the study group of 35 dyslexics and the total group are shown in Figure 4.1.

As we can see, the difference in average level of phonological awareness between the dyslexics and the total group is dramatic already a year before they start learning to read. This observation is important, because it tells us that phonological awareness is not only something that is developed by learning to read, but that it develops spontaneously through exposure to rhyming games, nursery rhymes, etc. before the child starts school. The dyslexic children obviously start their reading careers far behind the other students. Lacking the normal dose of phonological skills, their first exposure to reading and writing is bound to be difficult, and they risk winding up in a very vicious circle (Siegel, 1994).

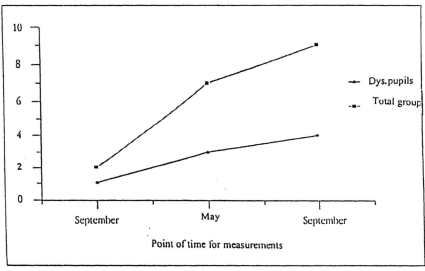

Figure 4.1. Phonemic awareness.
Average score at three points in time for dyslexic students (n=35) and for the total
group (n=395).

Part of this vicious circle can be seen in Figures 4.2 and 4.3, which show how the
dyslexic group and the total group did in grades one through three on tests of word
reading and writing. We see how the gap between the two groups grows bigger with
each measurement.

This study has shown that dyslexics have a much weaker phonological
awareness than normal readers, both during the year before they start school and at
the start of their schooling. Word decoding and spelling also show a poorer
development during the first three years of school. In this study we could not find
any other skill-deficit that could explain the dyslexics' reading and writing
difficulties.

Phonological Problems among Older Dyslexic Children

One might suppose that poor phonological awareness was only typical of very
young children with reading problems. Older, teenage dyslexics might have
overcome their initial deficit, but now be struggling with some other type of problem
at a higher level, for example with comprehension. The study we now present shows

that this is not the case (Høien and Lundberg, 1989a).

On the basis of an exceptionally precise selection procedure, 19 clearly dyslexic pupils were selected from a total population of 1250 cohorts. They were all 15-years old and in the 8th grade. Two control groups were formed, one of children the same age, but who read normally; and one consisting of younger students who were at the same level of general reading ability as the study group. (See Chapter 1 for the rationale behind using age-matched and reading ability-matched control groups.)

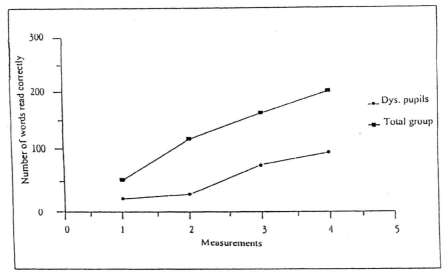

Figure 4.2.   Comparison of scores and reaction times on tasks of word reading, syllable reversals, and phoneme synthesis for dyslexics and two control groups.

All three groups were given a comprehensive series of tests. Most of the tests were administered on a computer, which registered both the number of correct/incorrect responses and the reaction time, that is, the number of seconds it took the student to answer the question or complete the task. This study yielded a wealth of data, but here we will only look at the results that have bearing on the question of phonological deficits among teenaged dyslexics.

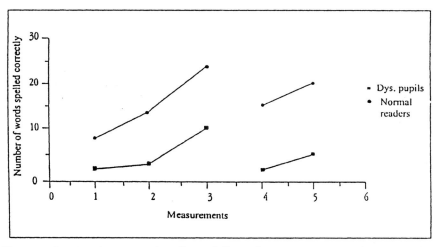

Figure 4.3. Development of spelling skills at five points in time during grades 1 through 4, dyslexics compared to total group.

The proportion of correct responses on the phonological tasks, and the reaction times on the nonword reading are presented in Table 4.2. We see that all the tasks were more difficult for the dyslexics. They even had a harder time than the younger readers, who were used as a control group precisely because they had the same general level of reading ability. Clearly, this tells us that the dyslexics' problem is rooted in phonology. Almost none of the dyslexics attained scores near even the weakest of the control students. In particular, the dyslexics managed to read correctly only a fourth of the nonwords, even though they used twice as much time.

Table 4.2. Comparison of performance in nonword reading, syllable reversals and phoneme synthesis for dyslexics as compared to two control groups.

Group		Reaction times (correct responses) nonword	Procent correct responses		
			nonword	syllable rev.	phoneme sythesis
Dyslexics	(N = 19)	3.18	76.8	63.1	68.9
Level-matched	(N = 19)	1.86	88.3	82.0	82.4
Age-matched	(N = 18)	1.43	94.3	90.7	91.1

The extreme length of the dyslexics' reaction times could be thought to reflect a generally slower tempo in answering all kinds of questions, not only in reading-related questions. To find out if this was the case, we measured their reaction times on various other types of tests. The dyslexics turned out to be somewhat slower than the controls, but this difference was not great in non-reading tasks such as visual comparisons, matching letters, naming objects, etc. In lexical decision tasks and in tests of rhyming their reaction times were much longer than the controls (Badian, 1997; Wolf, 1984).

On the basis of these results, we can confidently conclude that the characteristic trait of dyslexics, even when they are 15-years old, is a slow and inadequate phonological coding and a poorly developed phonological awareness.

We can therefore claim to have identified a specific deficit that dyslexics suffer from that is closely related to reading, but that does not seem to involve other domains in the cognitive system.

Compensating for the Specific Deficit

Other studies have also shown that phonological problems are common among older dyslexics (e.g. Bruck, 1992; Elbro, Nielsen and Petersen, 1994; Pennington et al., 1990). It is conceivable, at least in principle, that the teenaged dyslexics' phonological problems could be due to the simple fact that they haven't had as much practice reading or writing as their cohorts. Perhaps what we thought was the *cause* really was the *effect*, for indeed we do know that dyslexics don't like dealing with writing and that they avoid it as much as possible. Besides, there are some lucky people who had severe dyslexic problems in school, but who thanks to excellent teachers, a supportive home environment, and more than their share of true grit, have achieved an almost normal ability to read and write. We call them *compensated dyslexics*. The question is whether they still have their phonological handicap, or whether they have found techniques to get around their problem.

Gallagher et al. (1996) has studied well-compensated dyslexics who were attending college, and whose level of general reading ability was now within the normal range. They were compared to a group of normal readers (without any dyslexic symptoms) who matched the study group quite precisely in all other relevant ways. Gallagher found that the compensated dyslexics were clearly weaker than the control group in a series of phonological tasks. Particularly salient was the difference between the two groups in reading and writing nonwords. The compensated dyslexics were also much slower at dealing with spoonerisms and at reading numbers aloud. Their rate of speech was also slower.

This study dealt with talented people who had qualified for university education. Given their high level of general abilities, we may take them as evidence for the notion that the dyslexia deficit is sharply limited in scope and does not effect other intellectual functions. How these college students managed to compensate for their poor reading ability in primary school and ultimately achieve a fairly normal level of general reading ability is a question that needs more study. If we could understand more about the mechanisms whereby some dyslexics manage to compensate, then we would also know more about how to design remedial programmes.

Can Phonological Stimulation Prevent Dyslexia?

We know from many studies that phonological awareness can be boosted through stimulating games and exercises even in preschool. Bryant et al. (1989) have shown the importance of a stimulating home environment for the development of phoneme awareness. Olofsson and Lundberg (1985) and Lundberg, Frost and Peterson (1988) have shown how phonological awareness can be stimulated before the child starts school, even without teaching the letters. Children who are systematically encouraged to play with words, to find words that rhyme, to find as many words as possible that start with the same sound, to count the number of words in a sentence and the number of phonemes in a word, are shown to have a better start when they are start learning to read and write in school.

In the Danish study we presented earlier (Lundberg, Frost and Petersen, 1988), the children were divided into two groups, with approx. 12 preschools in each group. The study group, over 250 children, were given daily sessions with language games and exercises for 8 months. Children at the other preschools, the control group, were given standard Danish preschool training, which of course included a good deal of linguistic stimulation, but this was not as systematic or intensive as with the study group.

In the study group, the language sessions lasted around 20 minutes each day. The sessions were done in groups, and the children interacted in a lively manner. The games and exercises were arranged so that there were no 'losers' - everyone took part, and every child contributed. At the beginning of the 8-month period, the children were asked to focus their attention on the ambient sounds around them: birds chirping, cars driving by, etc. Gradually they started listening to the sounds of words. By working with rhyming games and nursery rhymes the children learned to move their attention from the semantic content of words - the point of communication - to the structure of sounds in the words. This is what they will need to attend to when they start learning to read and write.

The next step was to expand the focus to words and sentences. The children were taught what a sentence is, and how any sentence can be divided into a certain number of words. Then they were taught that words can have different lengths: some are as short as a grunt, while others run on for several syllables. An important exercise was to count out the number of syllables in a long word, and mark the number by clapping or stomping.

The next step was important. The children were asked to attend to the initial sound in words. The first words they were presented with began with vowel-sounds. This makes it easier to draw out the initial sound long enough for the children to latch onto it. Next they were presented with words that began with consonant-sounds that can be drawn out, s-, r-, l-, m-, n-, v-, and f-. The consonant stops, k-, g-, b- d-, p-, and t-, came last, because they are hardest to focus on. They were also given exercises in which they were given the initial sound and the sound of the rest of the word, and asked to blend the two to make the word.

After working on initial sounds, they started in on the final sounds in words. Here the consonant-stops could be presented earlier in the sequence. The final and decisive step was teaching a complete segmentation of words into phonemes, and the reverse, blending a series of phonemes to make a word.

When the children had learned to do these basic linguistic tasks, dealing with the alphabetic code is no insurmountable hurdle. The only thing they really have to learn in order to become productive readers and writers, is how letters code phonemes. When they have gained insight into how the system of writing functions - what the alphabetic code consists of - then children have the tools they need in order to start self-teaching themselves most of the rest. They are equipped to confront increasingly difficult types of texts, and make sense of them (see Share and Stanovich, 1995). But the preschool study did not go that far. In fact, we purposely did not start dealing with letters; doing so would have made it impossible to interpret the results of these children's later efforts at reading and writing, and it would have clouded the question we were trying to answer, namely whether it was possible to foster preschool phonological awareness without working with letters. In the real world, of course, there is nothing necessarily wrong with using letters in the types of preschool activities we have mentioned here. In fact, there are studies which seem to support the wisdom of doing so (Ball and Blachman, 1991; Bryant and Bradley, 1985).

Our study showed that specific training can cause children's linguistic awareness to make great leaps during the preschool year, in particular their ability to deal with phonemes. Children in the control group made almost no progress in phonemic awareness during this year.

The children's literacy development in school was studied several times. In general we can say that the systematic preschool training was valuable for most of the children. The study group's reading and writing went significantly smoother than the control group's. Linguistic training in preschool had clearly given the study group a 'softer' and more natural entry to written language. Cracking the alphabetic code was not a major obstacle for them.

How did the At-risk Children Fare?

We analyzed in particular the development of the at-risk children in the Danish preschool study (Lundberg, 1994). 50 children with very poor prognoses, 25 from the control group and 25 from the study group, were selected for his study. The selection was made on the basis of a test carried out at the beginning of the preschool year, before the language-training programme had started. To be selected for one of the groups, a child had to evince no sign of linguistic awareness on tests of rhyming, syllable counting, judging the length of words, identifying word-initial sounds, and the like. Their knowledge of letters was limited to one or two letters. They showed, then, no sign of 'reading readiness'. They also scored poorly on a vocabulary test. On the basis of earlier studies by ourselves and others, we had very good reason for judging them to be highly at risk for developing serious reading problems. We should point out, however, that the selection of children for this study was done *post factum*, after much of their of schooling was finished, at which time we went back and analyzed their earlier test-scores. Neither their teachers nor ourselves knew which of the children were at-risk when they started school. We wanted to find out whether at-risk children profited from their structured preschool training in phonemic awareness. We also wanted to find out whether the at-risk preschoolers who *did not* get the extra dose of training would, as we feared, go on to develop dyslexia. For purposes of comparison we also looked at the scores of the total group of preschoolers who did not get the extra training (the original control group). Figures 4.4, 4.5 and 4.6 show the results.

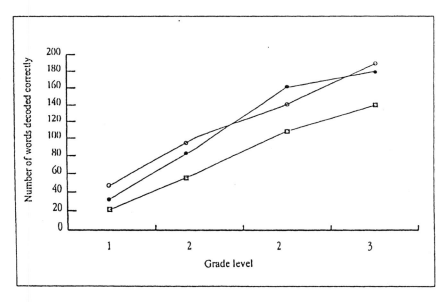

Figure 4.4. Development of word-decoding skill among at-risk children.
One group of at-risk children was given structured training during the preschool year, while another group of equally at-risk children was only given the usual, non-structured stimulation. These two groups are compared: (filled circle) at-risk children not receiving extra training, and (square) at-risk children who received the training. These groups are compared to (circle) all the children in the original control group, who did not receive the extra training.

In Figure 4.4 we see clearly that the at-risk children without the extra training are having problems decoding words. Throughout their first years of schooling, they seem to fall farther and farther behind. The at-risk children who received the extra training, however, are keeping up with the control group; their reading development is completely normal.

Figure 4.5 tells the same story with regard to spelling. Here we have followed the pupils all the way to grade 4. Because spelling ability always increases a lot during those years, we had to devise different tests for the different grade levels. In order to get results that could be compared, we converted the raw scores of the number of items spelled correctly to z-scores, which allow comparison. The horizontal line represents the achievement of the total control group of children who did not receive the phonological training. We see that the at-risk children without the training are always far under this norm, while the at-risk children who received the training swing a bit above the norm and then dip a little below it. In other words, their spelling ability is roughly comparable to the controls.

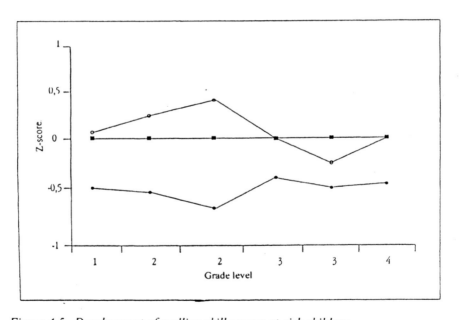

Figure 4.5. Development of spelling skill among at-risk children.
The results of at-risk children who received extra phonological training during preschool are compared to results of at-risk children who did not receive the structured training. Their raw scores are converted to z-scores, where the scores of the original control group are used as the norm. Three groups are compared: (filled circle) at-risk children who did not receive extra training, (circle) at-risk children who did receive the training, (filled square) all the children who did not receive the training.

The same pattern turned up when the children were asked to read sentences in the third grade (see Figure 4.6). Both times we tested their ability, in early Fall and late Spring, we found that the at-risk children without the training fared very poorly, while the at-risk children who received the training scored about the same as the control group. This indicates that they profited from their preschool exercises.

The high-risk children who didn't receive the training confirmed our original fears. They did in fact develop reading and writing problems, as we could predict from their test scores at the start of preschool. This confirms the claim that we can predict future problems for young children with poor phonemic awareness. This study also shows that it is possible in theory to remediate these problems before the children start school. But, again, we have to emphasize that our findings are valid at the group level. We have no reason to claim that *all* children would profit from extra training and stimulation at preschool age.

There is reason to believe that not all children are equally receptive for environmental stimulation and explicit training in phonemes. Some children do not learn quickly, and we do not have firm knowledge as to why this is the case. Variations among children in the ability to learn may have a genetic basis.

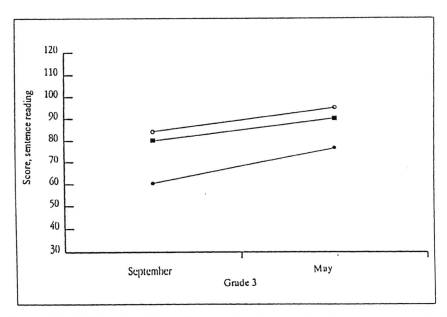

Figure 4.6. Ability of at-risk pupils to read and comprehend sentences in grade 3. Two at-risk groups are compared, those who received extra phonological training in preschool (circle), and those who did not (filled circle). Both groups are compared to all the children in the original control group, who did not receive the training (square).

Olson et al. (1989) carried out a large study of twins and rhyming. Their findings seem to indicate that genetic variation can explain a significant amount of the measured variation in the ability to perform rhyming operations. They also presented a behavioural-genetic analysis of word decoding data from identical and non-identical twins. Phonological coding during reading comprised most of the genetically conditioned variation, while orthographic coding was more conditioned by environmental factors (experience with words, teaching methods, etc.). In Chapter 6 we return to the question of genes and dyslexia.

Brief Summary

In this chapter we have looked at the special cognitive and linguistic demands that writing makes, and how these demands that are different than the demands speaking makes. Dealing with writing entails a degree of phonemic awareness, and dyslexic students do not seem able to achieve this linguistic insight. But studies show that explicit teaching of phonemes can, in many cases, prevent reading problems.

CHAPTER 5

DYSLEXIA AND READING COMPREHENSION

In the previous chapters, we have shown that the primary problems connected with dyslexia are at the word level. Decoding in reading and spelling are the big stumbling blocks. However, this does not mean that dyslexics have good reading comprehension. Most dyslexics do in fact have difficulty in understanding what they read. But these comprehension difficulties are usually secondary, a consequence of the poor word decoding. The slow, energy-demanding and deficient decoding makes such high demands on the reader's mental resources that there is no room left to carry out interpretation. If the dyslexic could be relieved of having to decode, for example by listening to a text being read aloud, one would expect good comprehension.

And in many cases this is what happens. But the reading comprehension of the dyslexic may be affected by other factors than decoding difficulties.

It is possible that the comprehension difficulties are not only a consequence of poor word decoding, but that the comprehension process is also directly affected by the phonological difficulties that are characteristic of the dyslexia problem.

Crain and Shankweiler (1990) maintain that difficulties with reading comprehension are caused by a combination of poor word decoding and poor listening comprehension. Skill in performing the tasks used to measure listening comprehension is not affected by word decoding ability, as here it is not a question of reading, but of listening to a text being read aloud. Even so, dyslexics generally score less well than normal readers of the same age in tasks based on listening comprehension. These authors explain this as a manifestation of difficulties with phonology, which affect both word decoding and the comprehension, and as the variance in reading comprehension depends on both word decoding skills and listening comprehension, phonological skills will play a decisive part in acquiring good reading comprehension.

Previous unsuccessful attempts at learning to read often have a serious effect on the dyslexic's self-esteem, his opinion of himself as a learning individual. He gives up, looses heart, and becomes passive. A passive attitude of this kind makes it more difficult to understand a text. As will appear from the remainder of this chapter, reading comprehension implies an active, constructive process, where the reader interacts with the text and makes use of his previous experience and knowledge. The passive reader has little chance of understanding the content of a text (Rayner, 1990).

    One reason why dyslexics have difficulty in understanding texts may be that they soon learn how to avoid reading. They seldom read spontaneously or voluntarily, never willingly or with pleasure. Reading is difficult and gives small dividends. It is like bicycling against a head wind. As early as in the second year at school, a normal reader may get through several hundred times as much text as a dyslexic. This means that the dyslexic gets far too little practice and familiarity with the written language and the distinctive characteristics of different text structures. In this chapter, we will take a closer look at reading comprehension and its relationship to cognitive attitudes, thus obtaining a better idea of the reason for the dyslexic's comprehension problems.

Reading Comprehension

In order to be able to read with comprehension, it is not enough to be able to decode words rapidly and automatically. In order to make progress with the interpretation of a text, *syntactic competence* is critical. But children's syntactic development is far from complete when they start school. They may meet syntactic constructions in writing that are very different from the language syntax they are familiar with. A simple and common example is provided by a construction of the type: 'John, the boy with the brown shirt, has a new ball'. When one listens to a pupil in the junior school battling with a construction like this, one realizes that writing makes new demands on children far beyond those connected with decoding. Here, knowledge of the form of language must also include grammatical structures.

    Many written sentences put great demands on short-term memory (also called working memory). The phonological problems of the dyslexic sometimes manifest themselves as a poor short-term memory. Information can effectively be retained in the working memory by coding it phonologically (Baddeley, 1986). Long sentences with complex syntax may thus be more difficult to cope with for a dyslexic with a poor short-term memory. Problems with attention and concentration may also enter the picture and further complicate matters for the dyslexic, even at the sentence level.

Vocabulary

In order to understand a text, it is important to be able to understand most of the words in it. If more than 20% of the words in a paragraph are unknown, one does not understand much of what one has read.

    There is reason to believe that many individuals with a dyslexic disposition have a smaller vocabulary than normal readers. There could be two reasons for this. In the first place, reading in itself plays a very important part in developing vocabulary. Most of the texts encountered by children contain more uncommon words than those met in conversation or in TV programmes. Those who read much are thus able to build up a rich vocabulary, which in turn encourages continued reading. The dyslexic's problem is that he/she tries to avoid reading. The chances of developing a good vocabulary thus decrease. This leads in turn to texts becoming unreasonably difficult, thus further strengthening the unwillingness to read. A vicious circle is thus established.

Secondly, it is possible that dyslexics' poor phonological competence also makes it difficult for them to learn new words. They have problems in remembering and recognizing them. They have to meet a word many times in order to master it reliably.

The phonological problems may be apparent as early as in infancy (Locke et al., 1997). When a child learns new words in the early development of language, the words are first handled as entities, i.e. as complete acoustic signals. However, as the vocabulary begins to contain more and more words, parsing becomes necessary, otherwise there is a risk of confusing words. A parsing principle thus implies that the words are built up of smaller units (phonemes) in accordance with certain rules. This is an important principle of information economy. A small number of units (only a few dozen) are sufficient to represent the endless richness of language (see Chapter 4).

Children with poorly developed phonological ability develop parsing late, which means that their vocabulary develops more slowly, and that their inner perception of how words are constructed is far too diffuse (Brady, 1997). Thus, we can see that the phonological problems that characterize dyslexia have different negative effects on word decoding and on reading comprehension.

Knowledge of the world

Word comprehension and syntactic processing are not all that is needed to understand a sentence. Primarily, the sentence has a semantic content. Consider this sentence for example: 'The policeman lifted his hand and stopped the car'. In order to understand the sentence it must not be taken literally. It is unlikely that the policeman can make the car stop by using his own physical strength. It is most probable that the sentence produces an image in the reader's mind, containing much information that is not given directly in the text. Images of this kind are often called scenarios. In the present example, it is assumed that there is a driver who steps on the brake pedal as a reaction to the signal given by the policeman with his raised hand. The reader makes use of his knowledge of the world - the role of the police in handling traffic - in order to develop an inner scenario. A completely different scenario is created by a sentence with the same syntactic structure, for example: 'The goal keeper lifted his hand and stopped the puck'. Here the scenario is based on knowledge of what might happen in an ice-hockey game. A text can be regarded as a series of instructions to the reader on how to use the knowledge of the world he already possesses, and how this knowledge can be modified and developed. In this way, reading becomes an active, creative process.

The reader always goes further than the information that is given explicitly, he reads between and beyond the lines, draws conclusions, or makes inferences. Conclusions of this kind also facilitate binding several sentences together. The following examples illustrate how sentences are bound together by means of conclusions: 'Lisa came flying down the stairs. Robert ran off to get hold of a doctor'. Here it would be possible to conclude that Lisa fell on the stairs and injured herself so much that Robert ran off for help. But there are probably many other possible interpretations, depending on the experience of the reader. One possibility could be that another member of the family had previously been injured or become acutely ill, and that Robert immediately understood how serious the situation was by the way Lisa rushed down the stairs. The reader thus goes beyond the information provided. A text that tells everything is terribly long-winded and boring. The writer should be able to assume that the reader is capable of drawing conclusions. The conclusions are sometimes rather subtle, as shown by the following example: 'Anna unpacked the picnic basket. The lemonade was hot.' In the second sentence the definite form *the* lemonade is an indication that information has already been given in the text. But there has been no explicit mention of lemonade in the text. The reader therefore has to build a bridge himself with a conclusion such as: 'Lemonade probably belongs in the picnic basket'.

Let us look at another example to illustrate the most important question of reading comprehension.

> Lena was on her way to school.
> She got off the bus two stops before.
> Later, she went to a café for a cup of coffee.
> She listened to some records in a shop, and took an automatic photograph of herself.
> She tried on some jeans in a newly opened shop. Later she went to the cinema.
> At four o'clock she went home again.

A simple text of this kind shows how much knowledge the reader has to have in order to understand the content, in addition to the information that is given directly in each sentence. The text contains much more than a sequence of facts, represented by written remarks. For example, most readers will understand that Lena is a school pupil, that she is supposed to be at school, that she is a teenager, and so on, although none of this is stated in the text. Many are also able to put themselves in Lena's position, they sympathize and commiserate with her, or they distance themselves from her and condemn her (Cain and Oakhill, 1999).

Background knowledge or previous experience thus plays an important part in reading. All readers know that it is easier to read a text on a known than on an unknown subject, even if the wording, grammar, and style are the same. The facts presented in a text are usually only fragmentary descriptions of situations and phenomena that are already known to us. A fruitful meeting between a reader and a text assumes that this previous knowledge is activated. Reading comprehension is thus an active, constructive process, an interaction between the reader and the text. If the reader does not have the relevant previous knowledge or prior understanding, the meeting is unsuccessful, irrespective of how well the decoding functions.

We can also regard the text as an invitation to the reader to activate an inner *schema*, a recipe or set of instructions that can help the reader to form an inner representation or a thought schema with categories into which the content of the text can be inserted or assimilated. The schema can be seen as an abstraction of experience that is constantly being brushed up and reconstructed in the light of new information received. Schemas can exist for objects, abstract ideas, performances, and occurrences. A prototype version of a situation or a fact is used to interpret the special incidents encountered in the text. This will also make it possible for the reader to go beyond the information given or to draw conclusions (Oakhill and Yuill, 1991, 1996; Carr and Thompson, 1996).

The schema also provides frames for interpretation and organization that improve information processing. It tells the reader when an episode in a story is over, it draws his or her attention to unexpected or divergent information. The schema is also used when the reader wants to remember what he or she has read. Many investigations have shown how the plans, motives, and properties that we attribute to someone in the text may have a drastic effect on our understanding of the course of events. The reader's perspective is also important. An investigation showed that when the reader was instructed to read a description of a house from the perspective of a prospective buyer, completely different details were examined than when asked to do so from the perspective of a potential burglar. If we are not able to activate a functional schema, the text becomes almost impossible to understand.

In recent years, research on reading comprehension has been aware of a special type of schema, *story grammar*, which specifies the underlying structures that appear in nearly all stories (Cain, 1996). A story usually starts with an introduction in the shape of an *outline* regarding time and place, continues with some kind of problem or *complication*, which is solved somewhere, and finishes with a *conclusion*. This simple, primitive structure can of course be expanded in different ways. In other words, a story can be schematized as a hierarchical structure around objectives and subsidiary objectives of the story, where the higher levels of the hierarchy consists of the *most important sentences,* and the lower levels consist of details and peripheral elements that do not help the story to progress. Several investigations have shown that the portions of text that are found at a higher hierarchy level are remembered better than the portions at a lower level. However, this effect is less clear in poor readers, indicating that they have more difficulty in differentiating between important and unimportant parts of the text.

The development of the story schema probably starts early, when children listen to stories being read aloud. All the stories have a common and recurring pattern that the children gradually and unconsciously experience as an organized schema.

Normally, the process of comprehension progresses smoothly and without problems. Inner scenarios are developed: conclusions are drawn that bind sentences together, signals are used in the text that facilitate binding together (e.g. small words such as *but, thus, since, afterwards*); pronouns and definite articles indicate what has been given already (references); special schemas are activated. All this happens more or less automatically and unconsciously, provided that the text is easy and does not contain any problematic items. More difficult texts require more active, planned, and conscious adaptation. It is then that the metacognitive sides of reading comprehension are relevant.

Metacognition

One important aspect of reading and reading comprehension is insight and awareness. The reader develops strategies and can make a conscious choice between different thought operations and different ways of getting started and surveying action alternatives. Such an attitude assumes that the reader becomes more aware of his own thought processes, that he can decide when he understands or does not understand, can steer and supervise his own learning and understanding, and choose solutions when problems arise. In recent years, researchers have shown a greater interest in these aspects of the cognitive processes. Metacognition has become a collective term for self-control and self-reflection on one's own thought processes, on one's own cognitive system (see for example, Craig and Yore, 1996).

In this section, we will look into the question of how metacognition and reading are connected. As we will see, metacognitive problems are present even in the beginner. We will examine parts of this, but above all concentrate on an analysis of metacognition in relation to reading comprehension and dyslexia at a later stage in the learning process.

Metacognition when learning to read

One of the first steps in learning to read is that the child does in fact realize that it cannot read. Pre-school children often have vague ideas of what reading really means. For example, they do not understand that the reader has to look at the writing and analyze the graphic information. An anecdotal example is the child that enters triumphantly with a much rehearsed fairy-tale book and says: 'Look, I can read without looking'. Downing (1979) is among those who have studied pre-school children's incomplete understanding of the concepts related to reading and writing. It has been shown that children arriving at school often do not understand terms like word, letter, item, row, top, headline, and page. Nor do they always know why we read, and what it means to learn to read. Lundberg and Tornéus (1978) showed that nursery school children even up to the age of seven years have vague ideas of the relationship between the correct length of the spoken and the written word. The child, who could not yet read, was shown a card with a couple of words written on it, for example *tree* and *tennis-racket*. The project leader told the child which words were on the card (with varied sequence from card to card), and asked the child to point to the word which says *tennis-racket*, and to state a reason for its choice. Many children could then point at the graphic picture for *tree* and explain its choice by saying that compared with a tree, a tennis-racket is small and therefore should have the short word. A child who answers like this is working from the word's semantic content and has not analyzed its shape. Some children pointed correctly and explained their choice by saying that it takes longer time to say tennis-racket than tree, and therefore that word should have more letters. These children had made a correct analysis of the shape of the word and were conscious of how the writing is related to the language, at least at a general level.

As we have seen, the great step for the person learning to read is to break the alphabetical code, i.e. to realize that the phoneme segments in the language are represented by graphemes. By no means all children who come to school have acquired sufficient linguistic awareness to be able to analyze the phonological structure of words. Phonemes are, of course, quite abstract linguistic categories which are not accessible to spontaneous perception. In the language, they are realized as co-articulated language sounds which can vary quite extensively depending on phonological context and situation. The child's natural attention is not directed towards the sound system either, but on the meaning and content of the message.

An important aspect of the initial process of learning to read is therefore to make discoveries, acquire insight and become reading-minded. The written word is found everywhere, on signposts and wrappings, in magazines, on TV, trains and buses, in shops. And even so, only a very small minority can break the alphabetical code on their own after many encounters with writing in everyday life. Most children, even those who learn to read before they start school, must be given methodical guidance in order to gain decisive insight. Learning to read is in many ways very different from learning to deal with oral language. Written texts are a «distant» communication form. Speech takes advantage of the immediate context the speaker and the listener share. Writing can't do that: words are written with the knowledge that they might not be read until sometime later, perhaps next year. Therefore, writing, in order to succeed, has to quite independent of context. This is one of the reasons children simply cannot «pick up» writing, like they pick up spoken language. Reading and writing have to be learnt, and they require a metacognitive attitude.

Learning to read is also one of the most important tools that the child can use to move beyond the limitations of his or her own experiences and everyday life, and to be able to reflect on language and on thought processes from a new cognitive level.

Thus, learning to read also covers development of general skills in self-adjustment and planning, which can be used in several different learning situations. However, the decoding operations gradually become more automatic, and function well without conscious effort. The metacognitive aspects of reading are then increasingly directed at the comprehension process.

Reading Comprehension and Metacognition

When we are faced with unknown material, we must frequently make a *conscious* effort in order to activate knowledge that can elucidate the content and the importance of the facts presented in the text. The reader must steer and supervise his understanding, discover faults and mistakes in his understanding of the text, and develop strategies that he can apply in order to correct the mistakes. It is typical of poor readers that they do not use active strategies of this kind when reading. They read passively, without self-regulating control of their own understanding. They are not able to notice and repair their faulty comprehension.

The first step, therefore, is to make a diagnosis of their own understanding, to discover problematic aspects of the text, to develop criteria for deciding whether they have understood the text or not. Markman (1977) showed that younger children (6-7 years) accepted instructions on how to play a certain card game, even though the instructions were incomplete and, therefore, totally incomprehensible. Older children (10-11 years), however, asked for more information to explain the obscure points. Harris et al. (1981) let children read a text which contained an irrelevant and unintelligible sentence. The text was read aloud by the child, sentence by sentence, and the reading time for each sentence was recorded. One text could for example be as follows:

At the hairdressers

John sits waiting.
There are two people before him.
Finally, it is his turn.
He notices how his hair gets shorter.
Luckily, there are no cavities this time
After a while he can get out of the chair
John puts on his coat again
He goes home and is pleased that it is over

One of the text lines is out of place (marked *). This line was read more slowly than the others by all the pupils. But the 11 year-olds were much better than the 8 year-olds at knowing which line was irrelevant. The slower reading was probably an unconscious adaptation to the peculiar character of the line, which was also noticed by the youngest readers. A metacognitive awareness is required in order to explain what the problem is - the youngest pupils appeared not to have acquired this yet. A failure to diagnose one's own faults in comprehension can be observed in many everyday school occurrences. For example, if a pupil in the fifth grade is asked to mention as many verbs as possible beginning with *s*, one pupil may respond with a general reaction which indicates total resignation. The pupil looks absolutely blank and states that he or she does not understand anything. Another pupil, more alert, cannot answer the question either, but asks: 'What's a verb?' This pupil at least knows what she doesn't know, and can ask for additional information.

In an investigation that was made at the medium level (Lundberg and Taube, not published), we let the pupils judge how easy they thought it would be to remember various sentences. Some sentences had a natural, logical structure with a certain continuity between the various parts, for example: 'The hungry man ate a large helping of pudding'. In other sentences, the parts did not follow each other equally naturally, for example 'The hungry boy at once lay down in the bed' or 'The man was very restless, and at once asked to be given a newspaper.' The pupils were given a long list of sentences, where sentences of both categories were mixed arbitrarily. They were asked to judge each sentence on a scale, and to indicate with a figure how easy or difficult it was to remember. A group of 40 pupils with reading and writing difficulties were compared with a matched control group of the same number of ordinary readers with the same result at Raven (a non-linguistic intelligence test). The result showed that those with reading disabilities noticed the differences between the sentences less often than normal readers. Thus, they have problems in analyzing the text, and cannot perceive different levels of demand. Therefore, they naturally have problems in adjusting their reading to the demands of the text.

A reader who discovers problems in the text or realizes his own lack of comprehension, can try to solve the problems by using *cognitive strategies*. It is typical for strategies that they are *consciously* chosen lines of action. One person chooses an activity more rapidly than another in order to reach a certain target. A well placed lob in tennis can be an example of a strategic action. But the lob could also have taken place through sheer luck without the player's conscious intention. In this case, the lob does not deserve equally strong applause. Thus, it is not the action itself that is strategic, but that the person shows a conscious intention. The use of strategies also means that they are available for introspection. This implies that the reader also can talk about them, discuss them, throw light on them. They can then be analysed and modified by the teacher. In training for sports, this is an important element. Strategies are thus the central aspect of metacognition.

Reading Strategies

All conscious and methodical control of activities that improves the chances of reaching a target, is part of a strategy. The reader's *target* also decides the choice of strategy. The purpose of the reading must be clarified, and the demands posed by the problem must be understood. Am I looking for specific information? Should I try to remember the main points in the story? Or is it a question of learning by heart? Steering and supervising the reading process is part of the strategic reading, thus enabling a decision to be made as to whether sufficient understanding has been acquired in relation to the original target. It may also be a matter of localizing the most important parts of a statement or a text, and of focusing one's attention on the main themes rather than on details.

The strategic reader tries to acquire a general impression first, by quickly skimming through the text. This is followed by re-reading certain parts of it, attempting to sum up the main content, testing comprehension by asking oneself questions, attempting to relate what has been read to previous knowledge, attempting to identify patterns in the text - how sequences of incidents are built up, seeking logical, causal, or time-related relationships, reading in advance in order to obtain clarity, leafing through what has already been read in order to check up, correcting when comprehension problems arise, and surmounting obstacles or irregularities that arise in the course of events. An *active* attitude like this marks the good reader. He or she has a repertoire of available strategies when problems arise and comprehension is endangered.

However, it is typical of many poor readers and dyslexics that they are *passive*. Somewhat exaggeratedly, we can say of poor readers: they cannot read clearly, they rarely re-read, they do not plan, do not take notes, and do not underline; nor do they attempt to express the content of the text in their own words, do not sum

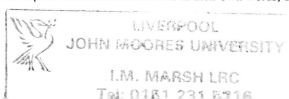

up, cannot distinguish between important and not important, and do not draw any conscious conclusions; they do not deliberately vary their reading speed, and do not realize that they do not understand. In weak readers, the lack of methodical self-control is striking. Before we try to understand this passivity, we should perhaps substantiate some of these observations in more detail.

In the investigation by Backman et al. (1984) mentioned above, it was found that the hierarchy effect was less pronounced in poor readers, which would seem to indicate that they had bigger problems than good readers with concentrating on important parts of the text and distinguishing between main and minor points. In the same investigation, it was also found that the reading speed of poor readers remained more or less the same, irrespective of the type of text they were given to read, and irrespective of how difficult the text was, while the good readers varied their reading speed by nearly 50 percent.

The poor readers' passive and non-selective attitude to reading was also evident in an investigation with a text concerning various types of boomerangs. Good readers noticed a little picture at the top of a page illustrating one of the two boomerangs described in the text. The eye movements disclosed that they used part of the reading time to look at the picture, while they were reading about the other boomerang, which had not been illustrated. They were obviously actively engaged in comparing the two types and in ascertaining what was the difference between them. The poor readers showed no signs of an active attitude like this.

The active reader also demonstrates ability to use both new and known information in a text to gain a better understanding of the content. In one investigation, certain words in a text were removed, either from the first or the last third of a paragraph. The task was to reconstruct which words had been removed. The paragraphs were constructed in such a way that the words in the last third could easily be reconstructed from previous text information, while the words in the first third could only be found if one read in advance or ahead in the text. Both good and poor readers could reconstruct the words in the last third, but it was only the good readers who managed the second alternative by reading ahead in the text. Good readers are more flexible, and able to make active use of the content of a text.

When we are faced with unknown material in a descriptive text, we must frequently make a conscious effort to activate knowledge which can clarify the content of the presented facts and what they mean. Take for example a pupil in the lower secondary school who reads a paragraph about blood circulation in the biology text-book. It says that arteries have thick walls and are quite elastic and transport blood with a high oxygen content from the heart. Veins, on the other hand, are thin and less elastic and transport blood with high carbon dioxide to the heart. To many pupils, such simple facts can seem arbitrary and confusing. Afterwards, they cannot remember whether it was the veins or arteries that were elastic. What was it that transported blood with a high oxygen content? Was it the thick-walled kind that transported blood to the heart? An active reader tries to see the given information in context with what he or she knows already, in which case it may be understandable that elasticity may be a good property when it comes to handling the blood that is pumped from the heart into the body. Poor readers may have the right knowledge, but not manage to activate it (Cain and Oakhill, 1998; Oakhill, Cain, and Yuill,

1998.

How can we understand the passive attitude of the poor readers, and the fact that they do not manage to learn reading strategies? First of all, we have to realize that it is a question of *cognitive economy*. To use strategies, we have to spend time and effort: mental resources are required. But such efforts should yield returns, for example in the form of richer and more interesting reading adventures, pleasure, progress, and clarity, a better way of reaching the target. The educational problem then becomes twofold: Firstly, we must guide the pupils so that they can use as effective and simple strategies as possible (economize with the resources staked). Secondly, we should give them a chance to reap the richest possible benefits from the resources (maximize the benefits). Thus, the pupils must be helped to be made aware of the limitations of their own information processing, and see how various strategies can be used to overcome the limitations, that something can be done about it. They should also realize that they can test themselves in order to find out whether they understand or not, and whether they should work harder or not. It is not enough just to learn a strategy, for example underlining or summing up. The strategies must mean something important to them as persons, become the property of the pupil, not just a way to please the teacher. The pupils must be given the chance to experience the positive effects of their own efforts deep inside them. As a concrete illustration of a successful attempt to break down the habitual helplessness of the weak pupils, we shall consider an example (Bransford et al. 1982):

> The pupils were given a list of sentences like the following:
> The kind man bought milk.
> The short man used the broom.
> The hungry man bought the tie.
> The bald man read the paper.
> The tall man used the brush.
> The fat man wrote a letter.
> The thirsty man opened the door.

When they had read through the list, they were asked to answer questions of the type 'Which man did X?' It turned out that it was only possible to remember a few sentences. The next step was to discuss why the material was so difficult to remember. It was pointed out that the relation between the various parts of the sentences was quite arbitrary. There was no logical or natural connection between, for example, being kind and buying milk. However, it was now possible, through an active and constructive effort, to produce a meaningful connection. The pupils were instructed how they could *build out* the sentences, analyze them. 'Why did the kind man buy milk?' The usual answer was 'because he was thirsty'. However, an analysis like that is not particularly precise. 'Even an unkind man may be thirsty. Any better answers?' Someone may suggest 'The kind man bought milk for the poor children'. Now we have a more precise analysis with possibly a somewhat strange, but even so reasonable relationship between the parts of the sentence. All the sentences are gone through in a similar way. Now the pupils experience the dramatic effect of the analyses. The whole material can be memorized. It is an exciting and happy experience. The pupils have learned to understand why one set of teaching material is more difficult than another. They have also learnt that they can have a certain control over their own understanding and their own thought and memory processes. We have thus shown them, through an example, that it is possible to break the habitual helplessness which characterizes pupils with reading problems to such a large extent.

We do not know much about the real background for such helplessness and passivity. It can of course be demonstrated that many pupils who are poor readers have a delayed general development, or a poor intellectual function. It is difficult to be aware of cognitive processes which one has not yet developed. But to characterize a pupil as backward is rarely of educational benefit to those responsible for providing remediation. When teaching, one should consider the interaction between at least four different components: 1) knowledge, hobbies, and interests of the individual, 2) available teaching strategies, 3) the nature and demand of the task, the target of the teaching, 4) the structure and content of the teaching material. Failure to succeed can be understood as being due to defects in the interaction between two or more of these components. To localize the cause of the lack in the individual is far too simple and unfruitful. A teacher who is alert, with a more open attitude, can prevent pupils from meeting serious defeats in their learning process, and can systematically guide the pupil towards an insight and awareness where the four components act harmoniously together.

Finally, we shall consider yet another side of the metacognitive development which was relevant in one of our investigations of poor readers in the fifth grade. When reading aloud a list of unrelated words, we found that some pupils made a quite bizarre mistake. When they failed to read a word, and this happened often, they quite quickly and without thinking made a quite wild guess which occasionally could be termed a poetical novelty. *Twenty-seven* could turn into *plenty of men*, *umbrella stand* into *upper grand*, *multiply* into *mull away*, and so on. One interpretation of this may be that, after a number of years in school with constant defeats, the pupils have learned that their own experiences, their own judgement, are quite without relevance in the school. School, to them, is a strange and confusing world, where you may in fact find *plenty of men* who *mull away*, even though the pupils have not themselves seen them. Because their own experiences do not count, they gradually learn not to think too much about what they read, and they no longer seem to have the inner criteria needed to appraise whether they are getting anything out of the text or not. Therefore, it is very much a case of the weak reader's self-esteem, his view of himself as a learning individual. We know from our own investigations (for example, Taube, 1988), that many poor readers have very negative self-esteem as early as in lower primary school. They do not believe in their own ability to learn, and lack the cognitive courage that is required when entering actively into a text. A reasonable hypothesis must be that metacognition and self-esteem are closely related, and in a characteristic way this may be expressed in the reading.

Brief Summary

In addition to syntactic competence, reading comprehension requires the development of inner scenarios, the drawing of conclusions, the utilization of text signals which bind sentences and paragraphs together, the application of schemas for organization and interpretation, etc. If the text is reasonably easy, and the content close to one's own knowledge of the world, interpretation takes place automatically and without effort.

Metacognitive processes enter the picture when problems arise. Thus, the first metacognitive problem is to know when one understands and when one does not. The next step is to choose cognitive strategies in order to solve the comprehension problem and reach the target of the reading. Strategic reading costs time and effort. The reader must receive a reasonable dividend on the resources that he stakes. It is typical of many dyslexics and poor readers that they are passive and non-strategic, they have a striking lack of self-controlled planning. Early learning defeats and poor self-esteem may lie behind this passivity and helplessness.

CHAPTER 6

THE BIOLOGICAL BASIS OF DYSLEXIA

Reading and writing are primarily cultural skills which are acquired as one becomes a member of the cultural community. Thus, learning to read and write cannot be compared with learning to walk or talk, which are more general, biologically based functions. No *normal* child can avoid learning to walk or talk. This has always been so, in all parts of the world. On the other hand, reading and writing are not natural functions. It is not until the present day, and in our part of the world, that the majority of people can read. But it is still estimated that 800 million adults in different parts of the world are illiterate. This is not because of cognitive dysfunction, but because they have not grown up in a culture that is based on written language.

Thus, if writing is primarily a product of culture, we cannot expect there to be a separate reading or writing centre in the brain, created by biological evolution, like the speech or motor centres. Even so, learning to read and write are, of course, based on fundamental biological functions such as visual perception, memory functions, phonological functions, and language comprehension.

In order to understand why some children develop serious reading disorders we must therefore also have a biological perspective. Naturally, cultural, social, and educational factors are often of critical importance when trying to understand why some individuals have an unsuccessful relationship to the written language. But there is much to indicate that individual biologically determined factors are also important. It is also not uncommon to find reading disorders in families which cannot only be interpreted as being due to social inheritance. Thus, genetic factors are considered to be very important in the aetiology of dyslexia. In this chapter, we will take a closer look at the results of research on the role of brain and genetic mechanisms in dyslexia.

Dyslexia and the Brain

Structure of the brain

Great steps forward have been made in brain research in recent decades as new imaging techniques have made it possible to study the brain in living people. The new techniques make it possible to see the structure of the brain, how it works, and which areas are active when the individual is faced with different tasks. Before going into the question of the relationship between dyslexia and brain function, we will give a brief description of the structure of the brain and its most important parts.

The human brain weighs just under 1.5 kilos. It contains about 100 billion different nerve cells, and each nerve cell is connected with thousands of other nerve cells. In other words, it is a system of enormous complexity. The cerebral cortex is the outer layer of the brain. Here we find almost only grey nerve cells. In other parts of the brain, there are numerous nerve fibres, which are surrounded by fat and contain nerve threads connecting the different parts of the brain with each other.

Roughly speaking, the brain can be divided into the cerebrum and cerebellum, each of which is divided into two halves or hemispheres (see Figure 6.1).

The cerebral hemispheres are connected with each other by numerous nerve threads that make up the *corpus callosum*. Almost every mental activity involves both hemispheres of the brain in intimate collaboration.

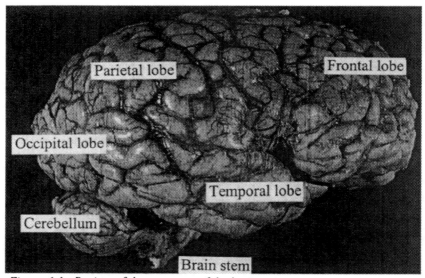

Figure 6.1.   Review of the structure of the brain.

The cerebral cortex can be divided into different areas or lobes (one in each hemisphere), which sometimes have different assignments. Furthest forward there are the *frontal lobes*, which are responsible for our conscious concentration, for planning, associating, and for inhibiting primitive impulses, etc. Furthest back there are the *occipital lobes*, one of the functions of these lobes being receiving and integrating visual impressions. Between the frontal and occipital lobes there are the *parietal* and *temporal lobes*, which are separated from each other by the sylvian fissure. Auditory impressions are integrated in the temporal lobes. The parietal lobes are involved with spatial information and make it possible to localize objects in the surroundings. Furthest back and furthest down is the *cerebellum*, which has primarily been considered as being responsible for motor coordination, control, and balance. In Figure 6.2 we have also marked two areas, *Broca's* and *Wernicke's* areas, which are important for our language functions.

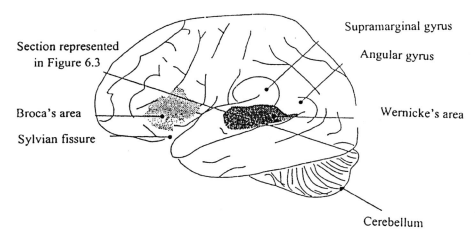

Figure 6.2. Lateral view of the left cerebral hemisphere.

Injuries to Broca's area on the left side may result in aphasia, making it impossible to produce speech. Broca's area is named after the French brain researcher, Pierre Paul Broca, who was active in the middle of the nineteenth century. He investigated people with aphasia after cerebral haemorrhage, and discovered that a limited area in the left frontal lobe (Broca's area) was necessary in order to be able to speak.

Injuries to Wernicke's area can lead to an aphasia that affects speech comprehension. This area is named after the German brain researcher, Carl Wernicke, who was active some years after Broca. One of the objects of his research was soldiers who had received brain injuries in the French-German war in the beginning of the 1870s.

In the region under the cortex between Broca's and Wernicke's areas there is a region called the *insula* (see Figure 6.3). This area is thought to coordinate the activities of Broca's and Wernicke's areas.

If the temporal lobe is seen from above from the sylvian fissure, one can see a triangular area called the *planum temporale*, which is also involved in language functions. The planum temporale is usually larger in the left than in the right hemisphere.

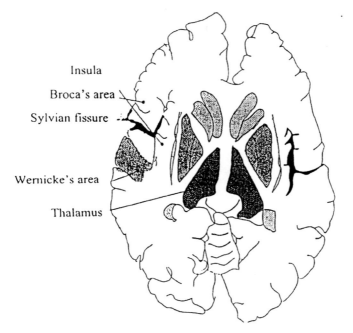

Figure 6.3. Horizontal section through the brain.

Insula

Broca's area

Sylvian fissure

Wernicke's area

Thalamus

In the interior, in approximately the middle of the cerebrum, there is the *thalamus,* which is an important station for relaying nerve impulses from the sense organs. The *lateral* and *medial geniculate bodies* are also here, which are involved in visual and auditory impressions respectively.

By studying individuals who have developed language disorders as a result of cerebral haemorrhages, it has been possible to increase the knowledge of the relationship between language and the brain. For example, it is now known that regions of the temporal lobe regulate some language functions. The *planum temporale* has been a special object of increased attention by researchers.

Studies of brain structure

Microscopy of brain tissue
This method is used to study the brain of deceased people. A direct microscopic analysis is carried out of the cell structure in different areas of the brain. This analysis makes it possible to demonstrate neurological deviations that might explain reading disorders (Galaburda et al., 1989).

MRI

MRI (Magnetic Resonance Imaging) is a method based on the fact that the hydrogen protons in body tissue emit energy when they are exposed to a magnetic field. These small energy impulses can be picked up by detectors and calculated in a computer. The result is seen as a distribution of dots of different light intensity on a TV screen, thus visualizing a cross section of the internal body tissues.

MRI is carried out by asking the patient to lie on a table with his/her head in a machine that resembles a space helmet. It is all very simple, totally painless, and completely without risk. The apparatus makes it possible to obtain pictures of successive sections of the brain. By studying a sequence of '*sections*' of the brain, it is possible to reconstruct the size of a brain area that is normally not accessible to direct observation (Courchesne and Plante, 1997).

The planum temporale symmetry and dyslexia

The planum temporale is an area of the cerebral cortex found on the upper side of the temporal lobes, within the sylvian fissure. Geschwind and Levitsky (1968) investigated 100 randomly selected brains and found that the planum temporale was larger on the left than the right in 2/3 of the brains, while the opposite was only found in about 10%. In the remainder, the plana were symmetrical. More recent investigations have shown that asymmetry, with the largest planum on the left side, occurs even more frequently than this (Galaburda et al., 1989). Weinberger et al. (1982) found that this asymmetry had developed as early as in the 20 weeks-old fetus.

In another series of investigations, Galaburda et al. (1987) studied the brains of eight deceased dyslexic individuals. These were all adults who had had obvious reading and writing problems both at school and later in adult life. In all eight cases, Galaburda found that the plana temporale were equally large on both sides. A unequivocal research finding like this is hardly due to chance. The statistic probability of this result being due to chance is so small that we venture to suggest that it is a most important finding. However, the crucial question is what this symmetry involves and how it should be interpreted.

First of all we must point out that symmetry does not mean that the planum is smaller on the left side than in normal readers. If it is assumed that dyslexia is connected with language disabilities, and that the left side of the brain is dominant regarding language, one would expect the planum temporale on the left side to be smaller than normal in dyslexics. Thus, symmetry would be established, as the right side is small already. However, this is not so. The size of the left planum temporale is normal, but the right planum is larger than normal in dyslexics.

Galaburda's investigation was on brains of deceased persons. In the Stavanger investigation (Larsen et al., 1990), we were able to study living brains using MRI (Magnetic Resonance Imaging). Figure 6.4 shows nine MRI sections of a brain. Picture 1 is furthest back towards the neck and picture 9 is furthest forward towards the eyes.

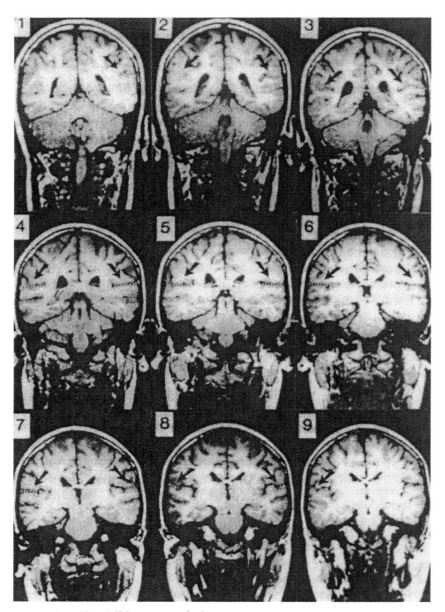

Figure 6.4. Nine MRI sections of a brain.

In each picture, the visible part of the sylvian fissure is specially marked and shown by an arrow. When we progress from back to front, the size of this area changes on both the left and right sides. Figure 6.5 shows how these markings are used to reconstruct a picture of the plana on both sides. The picture shows that in this case we have a brain in which the plana are about the same size.

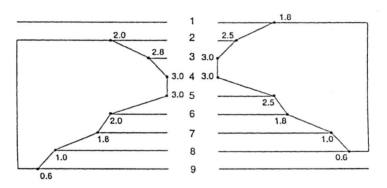

Figure 6.5. Reconstruction of the right and left plana temporale.
In this case the plana temporale in the right and left hemispheres are approximately the same size.

In the Stavanger investigation, there were 37 pupils from the 8th grade. They had been selected from a whole population of pupils at this level in Stavanger (N = 1250). 19 of the pupils were dyslexics according to a very strict definition (problems with word decoding and spelling, normal intellectual ability, no motor or neurological disorders, no socioemotional disorders). 18 pupils with normal reading skills for their age formed the control group. There was no difference between the control group and the dyslexia group as regards gender, age, intellectual ability, school environment, home environment, etc.

The main result of the MRI is shown in Table 6.1. Here it is shown how many asymmetrical brains were found in dyslexics compared with control pupils.

Table 6.1.   Incidence of symmetry/asymmetry in the planum temporale in dyslexics and normal readers.

	Dyslexia group	Control group
Asymmetry	6	14
Symmetry	13	4

We see that most of the dyslexics had symmetrical plana temporale, while, as expected, most of the pupils in the control group had asymmetrical plana. This is an interesting confirmation that Galaburda's findings in deceased dyslexics were correct. Symmetrical plana seem to be associated with dyslexia. For the first time, it was now possible to observe this in living dyslexics. A more interesting observation was that, in dyslexics, the asymmetry varied in relation to some characteristics of their reading problems. All the five dyslexics who had most severe phonological problems (nonword reading, phoneme parsing, phonemic synthesis) were shown to have symmetrical plana temporale. Most of those in an intermediate group of dyslexics with both serious phonological and orthographic problems also had symmetrical plana temporale, while the small number of dyslexics who did not have serious phonological problems tended to have asymmetrical plana. On closer examination of the control pupils, it appeared that two of the pupils with symmetrical plana did in fact have measurable problems with nonword reading and phonemic parsing.

What is particularly interesting in connection with the results of the Stavanger project (Larsen et al., 1990) is that it has been possible to observe a relationship between the result of a language-cognitive test and an abnormality of the cerebral morphology or structure. This is probably the nearest we have come to demonstrating a neurological basis for dyslexia (for a review, see also Davidson and Hugdahl, 1995; Hynd, 1997; Hynd et al., 1997; Riccio and Hynd, 1996).

Corpus callosum and dyslexia

The left and right hemispheres of the brain are connected to each other via thousands of nerve fibres that form the corpus callosum. If dyslexics have more nerve cells in the planum temporale on the right than on the left side, and thus a larger number of connections to the other hemisphere, one would expect that there would also be a larger number of fibres in the corpus callosum. In the Stavanger investigation, the corpus callosum was studied using MRI (Larsen, Høien and Ødegaard, 1992). But it was not possible to demonstrate a significant difference between dyslexics and control pupils. It is also not certain that the number of connections is directly related to the size of the corpus callosum. As will be known, the size could also depend on the degree of myelinization (to what extent the nerve fibres are insulated by fatty sheaths), or on how tightly packed the fibres are.

Cell structure and dyslexia

When Galaburda et al. studied the eight brains of deceased dyslexics, they also made other interesting findings (Galaburda and Kemper, 1979; Galaburda et al., 1985; Humphreys, Kaufmann and Galaburda, 1990; Rosen, Sherman and Galaburda, 1991). On microscopy of the brain tissue, they found curious deviations from the normal cell structure in some areas of the cerebral cortex. In all the brains they found curious wart-like accumulations of cells in the first layer of cortex, where nerve cells are not normally found. '*Ectopias*' of this kind were found spread over many areas of the brain, most of them on the left side, with an obvious concentration to areas round the sylvian fissure. Ectopias are only found in exceptional cases in normal brains, and then in very small numbers. The dyslexic brains usually had 100 ectopias or more.

Malformations of this kind cannot be observed with the present MRI technique. Nor is it possible to observe the '*dysplasias*' found by Galaburda in dyslexic brains, i.e. areas that lack structure in the otherwise well-organized column structure of the cells of the cerebral cortex.

It is likely that the deviations and malformations observed by Galaburda et al. in the dyslexic brains cannot have occurred as the result of injuries after birth. There is everything to indicate that they arose in the middle of fetal development, when the development of the nervous system is in its most critical phase. During a period of a few weeks, many billions of nerve cells have to be formed and find their place in a complicated architecture. When the process is at its most intensive, about half a million nerve cells are formed *per minute*. Every nerve cell of this kind has a fixed path to follow along finely woven threads, and has to reach a destination where it will send out axons and make connections with thousands of other nerve cells. Naturally, this extremely refined and precisely timed process can easily be disturbed by various factors. Both the hormone system and the immune system are assumed to take part in directing the formation, movement, and organisation of nerve cells. The ectopias and dysplasias found by Galaburda et al. in the dyslectic brains probably originate from disturbances in the early, dynamic phase of brain development in the middle of fetal life.

How can this be connected with the abnormally large right planum temporale in dyslexics? Here, we are still on uncertain ground; but some developmental biological reasoning is relevant none the less. A fundamental principle of all development is that the changes that occur are not only a question of growth and increase in size. Development is just as much a question of thinning out and selecting elements that do not function well enough or fail to compete. In this way, an inconceivably larger number of nerve cells are formed than the brain has use for. This thinning-out process starts already in the fetus. It is possible that cells from non-usable areas (e.g. in ectopias) on the left side have sent out axons and formed connections with cells on the right planum temporale. These cells on the right side have not been thinned out, but they still exist with connections far away in other parts of the brain. For a reason that has not yet been clarified, this abnormal structure of the dyslexic brain can lead to problems with certain language functions that affect the reading process. At the same time, it is possible that the abnormality can have some biological advantages: For example, it may make the brain less vulnerable to certain diseases or bestow upon its owner some measure of greater creativity in some fields.

In their investigations of the brain of dyslexic people, Galaburda et al. also found abnormalities in the subcortical regions of the brain, including the thalamus (Livingstone et al., 1991). The thalamus is the large relay station for sensory impulses from the sense organs. In the auditory area, the average cell size was smaller in dyslexic brains than in those of normal readers. This should mean that information processing was less effective and slower. In the visual system there are two types of cell: magnocells and parvocells. The magnocells handle rapid changes and movements. These cells were smaller in dyslexics than in the control pupils.

It has been shown in animal studies that the ectopias at the cerebral cortical level are connected with corresponding abnormalities of the thalamus. It has been found that some strains of laboratory mice also have ectopias in their brains and learning problems. In some way or another, the ectopias in the brain seem to block some functions. Ectopias have also been produced experimentally in rats. It is thus possible to study the nature and action of the ectopias in more detail (Rosen, Sherman and Galaburda, 1993).

On the other hand, environmental factors also influence neurological development. An animal experiment carried out by Schrott et al. (1992) demonstrates the complex relationship between biology and environment. She studied a special strain of inbred mice (New Zealand black mice), where there were many mice with ectopias in their brain, and they also had great difficulty in learning different tasks (e.g. finding their way in labyrinths, a task easily learnt by normal mice). She divided the mice into two equally large groups. One group was allowed to grow up under normal conditions for a laboratory mouse (a plastic cage with sawdust, a sloping water bottle). The other group was allowed to grow up in a larger cage with several mice in each cage, and with toys, ladders, mirrors, running wheels, etc. The mice that had grown up in the enriched environment were shown to manage labyrinth tasks just as well as normal mice without ectopias, while the other mice had exactly the same learning problems as one would expect in mice with ectopias.

We can conclude from this investigation that there is a plasticity of the nervous system that enables certain biological blockages to be avoided. In this case, it was obvious that the stimulating environment contributed to the development of compensatory mechanisms in the mice. It was not possible to remove the ectopias by environmental influences. The distance between mice and humans is naturally very large, and one should be careful to generalize.

An interesting aspect of dyslexia research is to investigate the relationship between deviant neuron patterns and reading problems. Are these cell deviations at the cortical level and in the thalamus the cause of the cognitive-linguistic problems of dyslexics?

As we have already mentioned, there are two types of cell in the visual thalamus (lateral geniculate body). There are parvocells in the four upper layers, and magnocells in the two underlying layers. Magnocells have specially obvious links with the cerebral cortex in the parietal lobe. Here there are special centres for localization of visual information, for spatial orientation, for visual attention, for peripheral vision, as well as for eye movements. All of these are of course important functions in reading.

It is therefore understandable that explanations of dyslexia have been looked for at the magnocell level (Livingstone et al., 1991; Stein and Walsh, 1997). Reference is made to perception experiments where it has been shown that dyslexics have problems in noticing small movements or perceiving certain patterns with broad stripes in poor light. But reference is also made to the findings made by Galaburda et al. in deceased dyslexics. In five cases, they found that the magnocells were more disorganized in the lateral geniculate body, and that they were on average 20 percent smaller. The thought behind the magnocellular theory of dyslexia is that the reading problems are caused by disturbances in very fundamental visual functions.

The starting point of Tallal's theory has been elementary auditory functions (Tallal, 1980; Tallal, Miller and Fitch, 1993). It has been found that children with language delays have more difficulty in perceiving rapid sequences of pure tones. Here it is assumed that the medial geniculate body in the thalamus plays a decisive part. In some brains from deceased dyslexics, Galaburda, Menard and Rosen (1994) found that the average size of nerve cells in the auditory thalamus was smaller than in normal control brains. These cells were thus thought to be the explanation of the problems with handling a rapid sequence of sound, which in turn would explain the phonological problems that are typical of dyslexia. In order to be able to identify a syllable of the type *da*, one must be able to follow the very rapid transitional flow of sound (40 milliseconds) that introduce the actual syllable. A complicated language disturbance is thus explained by an abnormality of a much more elementary function. However, an important question is whether the ectopias affect elementary sensory functions in such a way that higher functions are inhibited, or whether the opposite is true: that the higher functions in the cerebral cortex cause problems with lower functions.

Galaburda's cautious conclusion was that the causal direction may be the opposite, i.e. that a failure of the higher functions affects lower functions. We must still be content with speculations and hypotheses, but research on neurobiological development is now making very rapid progress. We can, however, note that studies on abnormalities of the brain cell structure in deceased individuals, who were considered to be dyslexics by their next-of-kin, have opened the way to a deeper understanding of the brain functions at a level that was previously unthinkable.

The cerebellum and dyslexia

After many years' research, Nicolson and Fawcett (1994a, b) maintain that the difficulties experienced by dyslexics in acquiring an automatic word decoding skill are caused by a defect in the cerebellum.

Large nerve pathways connect the cerebellum to the cortex. It is particularly important to know that the right cerebellum is connected with the left frontal lobe via a large nerve fibre. The left frontal lobe plays an important part in both phonological and articulatory language related tasks.

We refer here to two studies that support the theory that the cerebellum plays a more important part than previously assumed in the acquisition and performance of language skills.

In connection with the so-called brain bank (i.e. brains of deceased dyslexics), which has been established by the Orton Dyslexia Society, studies of the cerebellum have demonstrated interesting differences between dyslexics and normal readers. There were more abnormal cell structures in the cerebellum in dyslexics than in normal readers (abnormal neuron patterns in the visual thalamus and in the planum temporale, as well as the finding of ectopias).

In another study, researchers concentrated particularly on an area of the cerebellum called the *dentate nucleus* (Leiner et al., 1991, 1993). The dentate nucleus is an area that is particularly well developed in humans. The area is connected to the left frontal lobe via a thick nerve fibre. In humans, the dentate nucleus is important in connection with language activities. When this area is small, language problems are also found. For example, investigations carried out in autistic individuals have shown that they generally have a smaller dentate nucleus area than children in a control group. Children with autism, including those with normal intellectual ability, have communication and language problems. On the other hand, in children with Williams syndrome, whose speech development is normal but their general level of intellectual ability is low, the size of the dentate nucleus is normal (Leiner et al., 1991, 1993). An interesting object of future research would be to investigate the size of the dentate nucleus in dyslexics and hyperlexics. (Hyperlexics are those children - or adults - who decode words very fluently, and had no problem learning to do so, but who understand very little of what they read.)

It is also interesting to note that the nerve connections from the cerebellum to the cortex run via the thalamus. We have already mentioned the role played by the thalamus in processing visual and auditory stimuli (Livingstone et al., 1991).

The cerebellum also plays an important part in the acquisition of both motor and language skills. From time to time, the question arises of the relationship between motor and reading skills. Are these two skills causally related to each other?

Good motor skills are of course important in themselves, and they are also needed for both writing activities and articulation, and for the development of good self-esteem. Good self-esteem is important in turn for all learning, including learning to read. In this respect, it can be said that good motor skills are important in order to learn to read. But this gives an indirect causal connection between motor skills and reading. The controversial question is whether there is also a direct connection between motor skills and reading.

A couple of studies have been carried out recently which may help to throw more light on this question (McLagan et al., 1997). McLagan et al. (1997) found that balance training had a positive effect on the development of reading and writing skills. In another study on children with learning disabilities, Nicolson et al. (in print) found that balance training increased the verbal IQ compared with a control group. They therefore recommend that balance training should be included with phonological training in the programme for so-called risk pupils and dyslexics. However, one should at present be careful to draw too definite conclusions, but rather wait for further research in this field. Until shown otherwise, we strongly maintain that reading training gives better results than motor training if the object is to improve reading skills. Some counter evidence for the balance-hypothesis have been reported by Wimmer, Mayringer and Raberger (1999).

The brain in action

So far, we have described two different ways of studying the brain in connection with dyslexia. One method entails analyzing the brains after death by direct observation of anatomical and morphological conditions, or by microscopy studies of the cell structure. The second method is MRI, which can be used in living individuals without risk. Both methods aim at understanding the structure of the brain. However, it is just as important to study the brain in action, how it works and is activated when different tasks are performed, for example reading and writing.

EEG and BEAM
The classical method of studying the brain in action is EEG (electroencephalography), where the weak electromagnetic impulses arising from the activity of the nerve cells can be picked up by electrode plates on the skull and be amplified. The activities from different areas of the brain can be studied as curves on a sheet of paper, where the rhythm and frequency of the curves provide information about the level of activity. However, it is not easy to interpret and compare all these curves merely by looking at them.

In recent years, a number of computer-based methods have been developed, where a colour diagram allows us to see how the activity varies in the different regions of the brain. One such method is called BEAM, which stands for Brain Electric Activity Mapping.

PET
A study of the brain *in action* is often based on the blood circulation in different parts of the brain. It has been found that there is a close relationship between the amount of blood that is circulating in an area and the neural activity taking place there. With the *PET technique* (Positron Emission Tomography), the blood circulation is measured by injecting radioactive water labelled with an oxygen isotope. The labelled water, which emits positrons with a half-life of about 2 minutes, accumulates in the brain in less than one minute. Using detectors that pick up positron emission and a computer that can transform information into comprehensible colour pictures, a clear representation of the blood circulation in the brain is obtained, and thus also the neural activity that occurs while the positrons are being emitted. In a PET investigation the test subject places his/her head inside something that resembles a large helmet with detectors placed in different positions on it. Different tasks can be presented to the person being examined, on a screen or through headphones, and changes in the brain activity pattern can be studied as the

tasks change.

fMRI

A new technique has been developed in recent years that does not involve radioactive labelling. It thus becomes possible to examine younger individuals with dyslexia as well. The technique is called fMRI (functional Magnetic Resonance Imaging) and has a more complicated relationship to the blood circulation in the brain. It is based on the fact that when the blood circulation increases with increase in brain activity, the amount of oxygen used does not increase. There will then be more oxygen locally in the tissues, since the circulation (and thus the oxygen supply) has increased, while the need for and the consumption of oxygen have not increased. The amount of oxygen in the haemoglobin molecules of the blood affects the molecule's magnetic properties. This can be made use of because detectors can pick up changes in a magnetic field.

In fMRI as well, the test subject puts his/her head into something that resembles a helmet covered with detectors. But now a magnetic field is also introduced. No negative side-effects of having one's head in a weak magnetic field are known, which means that fMRI may become an important tool when investigating children with dyslexia.

In both PET and fMRI, the investigation starts with a control situation, for example the test subject just looks at a fixation point on the screen (see Raichle, 1994). Then a task situation is introduced, for example looking passively at written words without trying to read them. By comparing the pattern of the blood circulation in the two situations, it is possible to discover which regions of the brain are particularly active during the task. In the control situation in this case, the visual centre in the occipital lobe of both hemispheres is activated. In the task situation when words are exposed below the fixation point, additional regions of the brain are activated. The next step consists of the test subject reading the words aloud. Then there is also activity in motor areas, in the cerebellum, and in the areas round the sylvian fissure (which separates the temporal and parietal lobes). It is interesting to note that both the hemispheres are activated when reading words aloud.

In the next step, instead of reading a word, the test subjects were asked to suggest a verb that fitted the word: for example the verb *to cut* fits with the word *knife*. Now some activity was also seen in the frontal lobe area and some further to the left in the more traditional language areas (Broca's and Wernicke's areas). Areas in the right half of the cerebellum were also activated (Shaywitz et al., 1996).

Other techniques

One disadvantage of PET and fMRI is a certain sluggishness. Another disadvantage of fMRI is that it may be too sensitive and thus measure irrelevant 'noise'. It is not possible to pick up very fast events. As previously mentioned, classical EEG (electroencephalography) consists of studying the brain activity by picking up weak electromagnetic impulses by electrodes placed directly onto the head. The impulses can be amplified and processed and are recorded on graphs which show the waves from different parts of the brain. The rhythm and frequency of the waves provide information on the level of activity. Here the time relationship is good, but the spatial precision is poor.

One variant of EEG is the ERP technique (Event Related Potentials), where the individual is exposed to repeated stimuli at the same time as an EEG recording. The fact that the stimulation occurs repeatedly, makes it possible to record the brain's response to stimulation on a computer, as all irrelevant 'noise' is removed from the recordings. The waves that remain provide interesting information on the brain activity.

A new variant of EEG is called MEG (magnet encephalography), where changes in a magnetic field can be picked up and processed. Here the time relationship is the same or better than with EEG, and the spatial precision is slightly better.

Is the brain activity different in dyslexics?

Wood (1989) has shown that the PET pattern (a coloured map of the level of activity in different regions of the brain) is more distinct in dyslexics than in normal readers, and that it contains several marked, well-defined areas of increased activity. Obvious differences in activity are seen specially in deep regions of the temporal lobe on both sides of the brain in dyslexics. We do not know yet whether this is connected with symmetry of the planum temporale. Like BEAM, the PET technique also shows that the activity in the frontal lobes is different in dyslexics.

Duffy (1989) has compared the activity curves in dyslexics and normal readers during reading. The BEAM diagrams were then put on top of each other and a computer calculated the mean difference between the groups. A difference diagram of this type clearly shows that the main difference between dyslexics and normal readers is found in the temporal lobe when they read a text. But there are also significant differences in the so-called prefrontal motor areas in the frontal lobe. It was found that the prefrontal areas were underactive in dyslexic boys when they were engaged in cognitive tasks. It is possible that this prefrontal difference reflects varying ability to concentrate.

When the brain activity is compared in dyslexics and normal readers, several differences will probably be found. Interpretation is, however, problematic. Do the differences really mean that the dyslexic brain functions in another way? The task of reading words is considerably more difficult for dyslexics than for normal readers. The differences in brain activity may then be a result of varying degrees of difficulty.

In an investigation carried out by Paulesu et al. (1996), an attempt was made to avoid this problem by studying adults (university students) who had compensated for their dyslexia. They had encountered great reading difficulties early in school life, but by good special education, good support at home, and hard work they had overcome their problems and were now able to read almost normally. The question was whether their previous dyslexia still had any effect when they were faced with phonological tasks.

Both normal readers and compensated dyslexics were given simple rhyme and short-term memory tasks during PET scanning. In the rhyme task they were presented with a couple of letters (for example *B* and *T*, or *D* and *F*), and by pushing a button the test subject had to say whether or not the pair rhymed. In the short-term memory task they were presented with a series of six letters. After this, a single letter appeared and the question was whether this letter had been among the previous series of letters. Both tasks were so easy that the dyslexics generally replied correctly to all the questions. But even so there were differences between the groups in how the tasks were performed.

In order to solve the rhyme task, one has to produce an inner sound image of how the letters sound and parse the names of the letters so that the same vowel-sound is obtained in *B* and *T*. In the memory test, one has to decide whether one had seen a letter before. Here it is likely that the test subjects repeat the names of the letters silently to themselves as they are presented. In both the rhyme and the memory tests, control tasks were given that did not require any inner sounding out. Unpronounceable visual symbols were used (Korean logographs).

The differences in brain activity between the phonological and the purely visual tasks were very obvious. The phonological tasks activated the areas round the sylvian fissure in the left hemisphere (including Broca's and Wernicke's areas, the insula and the lower side of the parietal lobe). In normal readers, all these areas were activated simultaneously. In the compensated dyslexics, the activity in the *insula* was obviously reduced, indicating a poorer connection between the anterior (Broca) and posterior (Wernicke) parts of the language system in the brain. Although the dyslexics managed the phonological tasks just as well as normal readers, their brain activity pattern was different. Paulesu et al. (1996) interpreted this as evidence that dyslexics had difficulty in carrying out inner sounding out, and that they therefore performed simple phonological tasks in a different way from normal readers. One explanation could be lack of activity in the insula region. According to these researchers, dyslexia may thus be a question of a disturbance in the connections between different language areas which makes information processing difficult for the phonological module.

The part played by the cerebellum in connection with reading has also been investigated using fMRI and PET. Raichle (1994) studied brain activation in a patient with damage to the cerebellum. After the brain injury, the patient found it difficult to read. A characteristic of the reading was that the patient was not able to see his own reading errors. He also developed motor problems. Therefore, Raichle concluded that the cerebellum was responsible for more than just motor control and coordination, as had previously been thought. These findings were supported by Paulesu et al. (1996), who mapped brain activity while various language tasks were being performed. They found that there was clearly less activation of the right cerebellum in dyslexics than in normal readers during reading. They also found reduced activity in the cerebellum of adult dyslexics during motor tasks compared with normal readers.

Techniques for measuring the electrical activity of the brain and the blood circulation during cognitive and language activities are now being developed at a rapid pace. It should therefore be possible to obtain more knowledge of the structural and functional deviations in the nervous system of dyslexics. It is believed that biochemical factors play an important part here.

The nerve cells relay information as electrochemical impulses. But in order to communicate with each other, cells have to pass the signals through *synapses*, the connections between the nerve cells. The messengers between cells over synapses are called neurotransmitters. Many substances influence the neurotransmitter effect either by preventing the nerve cells from taking up the transmitter substance or by increasing its effect.

There is reason to believe that, behind the brain functions that can be observed by various techniques, an important part is played by neurotransmitters and other biochemical substances. Current research aims at finding out to what extent the neurological differences found in some dyslexics could be due to variations in the amount of and balance between these biochemical factors (for an overview see Duane and Gray, 1991; Galaburda, 1993; Hugdahl, 1995).

Dyslexia and other biologically-based disturbances

Recent research on dyslexia has also looked at the co-morbidity of dyslexia, i.e. to what extent dyslexia occurs simultaneously with other developmental disorders (Hertzig and Farber, 1995). Special attention has focused on the relationship between dyslexia and ADD problems (Ackerman et al., 1994; Duane, 1999), dyslexia and ADHD (Pennington et al., 1993), and dyslexia and autism (Knivsberg, 1997; O'Connor and Hermelin, 1994). An increased frequency of immunological disorders (e.g. allergy and asthma) has also been found in dyslexics (Geschwind and Behan, 1982, 1984; Geschwind and Galaburda, 1984; Hugdahl, 1993; Tønnessen et al., 1993).

Some teachers, when confronted with the hard neurological facts described in this chapter, may want to give up: If the pupils' problems have a clear neurological basis, then what can I do about it? We cannot and do not agree with such a pessimistic conclusion. As we have repeatedly pointed out, reading is a culture activity which needs to be taught and trained. Some pupils need *more* teaching and training, and sometimes even *different* teaching and training. For biological reasons, learning may be more demanding for some people than for others. The teacher should take this as a challenge to instruct, stimulate, and teach even better. Those who have a biological handicap to overcome need even more support, guidance, encouragement, and training. Only in very, very extreme cases are the biological obstacles so great that teaching becomes hopeless.

Dyslexia and Inheritance

Genes are responsible for inheritance. There are about 100,000 genes and about 10 trillion cells in the human body. In each cell there is a cell nucleus. Each cell nucleus contains 23 pairs of chromosomes in which the genes are stored. One of the chromosomes in each of the 23 pairs contains genes from the father and mother. The chromosomes consist of tightly packed DNA molecules that together make up the genome. The genes are the parts of DNA that contain instructions to produce protein, of which the body is built.

When it is maintained that dyslexia is inherited, it is important to stress that it is not dyslexia in itself, but the genes that are inherited. In the cells' chromosomes, there are a very large number of genes that steer the synthesis of amino acids. In this way, genes decide our abilities and talents. They also affect how we react to influences from the environment. Reading is based on culture and cannot be directly affected by genes. However, we have seen in earlier chapters how basal functions such as memory and concentration can affect reading skills. Genes determine the development of the nervous system, which in turn affects how these abilities function. This is only a brief outline of the possible connection between dyslexia and genetic disposition.

Figure 6.6 is an illustration of the interaction between inheritance and environment as regards dyslexia.

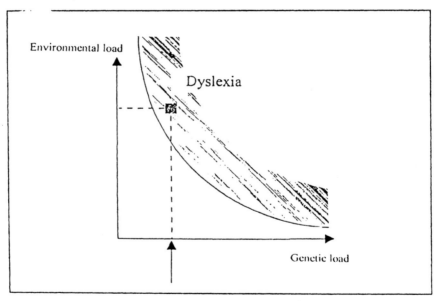

Figure 6.6. Interaction between inheritance and environment.
If the hereditary disposition is small (see arrow), much worse environmental conditions are needed before dyslexia appears.

Genetic research differentiates between phenotypes and genotypes. A phenotype is the collection of symptoms and characteristics that are distinctive or characteristic of a phenomenon, in our case dyslexia. The genotype is the genetic basis of this phenomenon (Pennington, 1997).

Although a genotype cannot be observed directly, it can be defined.

Phenotype on the other hand can both be observed and defined. Genetic studies generally start with the phenotype in order to find the genotype. However, there could also be cases where the genotype is known and it is desired to find out how just this genotype is expressed as a phenotype.

The distinction between phenotypes and genotypes also explains why people with similar genetic inheritance often have very different levels of achievement. In the same way, people with the same level of achievement may have different genetic make-ups. This is an example of the interaction between inheritance and environment. Genes give the child a disposition, a personality, which determines how receptive the child is to stimuli in the environment. But the child is also an active and constructive being who makes choices in the environment and decides which experiences he wants to make. The child also affects his environment, he influences the adults so that they treat him in accordance with his personality. The child is thus not a passive recipient but an active creator of his own environment. He chooses from the environment, hunts for niches, and influences the environment.

Children with a personality that makes them particularly receptive to verbal stimulation generally ask someone to read to them. They make an active effort to seek the world of books, influence the parents so that they are given books for Christmas and birthday presents, stimulate the parents to tell stories, take them to the library, etc. Children with language problems may talk so incoherently and incomprehensibly that the parents usually give them non-verbal signals. These children do not sit for long on a lap listening to someone reading aloud, they slip away and do something else. They seem almost deaf to nursery rhymes, etc. Should one accuse the parents of doing a bad job in such cases? Perhaps the child's personality makes it an active participant in this process? Poor reading skills in children when they start school may be partly due to less-than-natural talent for language activities. Learning to read puts these talents to a hard test.

The most important arguments in support of genetic basis of dyslexia

1. Family studies
The classical argument in support of dyslexia being hereditary is of course the high frequency of dyslexia found in some families. However, it is often difficult to obtain an exact picture of the environment or of the cultural and social conditions present in different families. If several generations are to be investigated, collection of information from the oldest generation is specially problematic. For example, compensation and reduced health can deflect the results in opposite directions. Misleading recordings of this kind make it difficult to compare with younger generations. Another reason why this comparison is problematic is that written language and reading skills have a completely different significance today than before. Today it is easier both to have reading training and to discover reading problems. It is also clear that today's school system provides better basic teaching and better remediation. Therefore, when the oldest generation is interviewed about earlier reading problems, a misleading picture is not only due to lack of honesty or failing memory. Completely different conditions for growing up may make

interpretation and comparison of information very difficult.

A major investigation in Colorado has been the object of most interest in connection with the assessment of the occurrence of dyslexia in families (see for example DeFries et al., 1985). In this investigation, the relatives were also tested with an extensive battery of reading and writing tests, and with different linguistic and cognitive tests. A total of over 1,000 people were investigated. Several genetic models were tried. The so-called polygenetic threshold model has been the object of special attention and interest. It was assumed that a combination of inheritance and environment was responsible, and that several genes determined the inheritance. The threshold model implies that individuals who come over a certain threshold value develop manifest problems. This threshold is thought to be higher in girls than in boys, so that the genetic load has to be higher before girls develop dyslexia.

Another strategy for family studies on reading problems was carried out by Lundberg and Nilsson (1986). They investigated many generations of poor readers by using Swedish church registers. Using a five-fold scale, they recorded how well the members of the parish read aloud. Recordings of this kind had been made as early as the 18th century, long before compulsory schools were introduced. Many people underwent several reading tests in the course of their lives. The tests were often performed by different priests. Those who were consistently given the lowest marks can probably be said to be genuinely poor readers.

17 very poor readers were selected from a very large sample. An equally large group of good readers from the same social level was also selected. The two groups were investigated and compared over several generations. The results showed that reading skills had a clear tendency to be inherited. However, the investigation did not provide evidence to enable conclusions to be drawn on heredity or genetic mechanisms.

In another family investigation (Høien et al., 1989) of 19 well-defined dyslexic pupils in the 8th grade, dyslexic symptoms were found in the closest members of the family in 13 cases, and in near relatives in 3 cases. Only 3 cases of dyslexia were found in the families in the control group of normal readers. So far, this investigation confirms earlier results. A more striking finding was that when the fathers or mothers of the dyslexic pupils were tested using an extensive battery of word and phonological tests, it appeared that their profile was more or less the same as that of their children, though the parents' achievements were often at a higher level. The phonological deficit was particularly obvious in both children and parents. If these results also appear in later investigations, this would be a good indication that there is a hereditary component in dyslexia. The result could also contribute to a better definition dyslexia's phenotype.

2. Twin studies

Twin studies have also had a central position in the argumentation for dyslexia being hereditary. Monozygotic (identical) and dizygotic (non-identical) pairs of twins are selected in these investigations. The principle behind the studies is that monozygotic twins have identical genes while dizygotic twins do not have more genes in common than normal siblings. If both members of a monozygotic pair have reading problems much more often than both members of a dizygotic pair, it is considered that this must be attributed to the genes they have in common. These investigations have generally found differences between mono- and di-zygotic twins, but there is disagreement on how large or how significant the differences are. Among recent investigations, we can look specially at that carried out by Decker and Vandenberg (1985), who found that 85 percent of the monozygotic and 55 percent of the dizygotic twins had a joint diagnosis. Most of the earlier investigations have found a slightly larger difference between the two groups. For example, in his classical investigation, Hermann (1959) found a joint diagnosis in 100 percent and 33 percent respectively.

Based on twin studies, Olson et al. (1989) have estimated that reading problems were about 40 percent due to inheritance, and about 60 percent due to environment. They maintain that phonological coding or the ability to parse sounds is more strongly linked to inheritance, while orthographic coding is mostly influenced by environmental factors such as teaching methods and reading stimulation. This result provides further support for our hypothesis that phonological defisits are dyslexia markers. *Inter alia,* the Colorado investigation has shown that, in the youngest pupils, the word reading skills are the most hereditary aspect of linguistic abilities. In some older pupils (over 11 years), it was spelling that was most hereditary (DeFries et al., 1997). This seems quite reasonable, as a poor word decoding skill can be compensated for by using contextual cues. Poor spelling, on the other hand, is more difficult to compensate for in the same way, in the long term.

One question raised by twin studies is how large the differences between the two types of twins has to be in order to make it probable that inheritance is the most likely explanation. For example, it should be taken into account that monozygotic twins will probably be influenced in the same way by the same environment. On the other hand, if both of the twins in a dizygotic pair grow up in the same environment, it is less likely that they will finally have the same characteristics and abilities. With different genes, they will probably be influenced in different ways by the same environment.

Although we should demand of a study that the environment is roughly the same in both types of twins, this still would not be sufficient to establish the relative importance of inheritance and environment. We should also note that the samples were often small in the twin studies. This applies particularly to the monozygotic twins. How can one know whether they are representative? Perhaps a larger sample would show a larger number of monozygotic twins who did not have a joint diagnosis.

Stevenson et al. (1986) also think that the age of the twins can influence the results. After an investigation of 285 pairs of twins of 13 years, they conclude that, at this age, genetic factors only play an insignificant part in reading problems. If this is correct, it is clearly important that the different pairs of twins in any one study are about the same age. However, Olson et al. (1989, 1990) doubt whether so much importance can be attached to age. Although twin studies involve certain methodological problems, they have obviously been able to throw new and important light on the question of inheritance and dyslexia. Olson et al.'s (1997) demonstration of how different components of word reading have a different genetic basis is extremely interesting.

3. Dyslexia persists

A third factor in favour of hereditary factors behind dyslexia is that reading problems are often difficult to remove by environmental, educational, social, or cultural intervention. Dyslexia has a tendency to persist throughout the whole life of many (see the section 'Prognosis of pupils with dyslexia' in Chapter 8). There is of course some disagreement on how much reading problems can be influenced by remediation. To a certain extent, compensatory reading strategies can be taken into use, thus reducing the handicap. The tendency of dyslexia to persist indicates that there is a constitutional or biological background to the condition. However, before attributing this to genetic causes, one must exclude possible injuries during pregnancy, birth, or childhood. It can be pointed out here that Owen (1978) did not find that children with learning and reading problems had been exposed to more injuries than others. This result therefore points in a slightly different direction than earlier investigations, where a high frequency of premature births was found in dyslexics. A larger number of disorders, diseases and/or other problems before, during, and immediately after birth were also found.

Although it is not possible to demonstrate early injuries in dyslexics, like those mentioned above, this does not exclude the possibility of a genetic disposition that produces susceptibility to extreme environmental stress, and also predisposes to difficulties in learning to read.

4. Higher frequency in boys

A higher frequency in boys than in girls (see for example Critchley, 1970) could also point towards a hereditary element. Although it is usually assumed that there are three to four times as many dyslexic boys as girls, it should also be mentioned that some researchers consider that the difference is insignificant. For example, Hallgren (1950) found no special difference. He considered that the large differences previously recorded were because the boys' problems were given more attention than the girls'. By and large, this reasoning agrees with findings made by Vernon (1957).

Sex hormones may contribute to another explanation of possible differences between the sexes. Geschwind's (1985) hypothesis on the effect of testosterone on lateralisation and dyslexia can be mentioned as an example here. Another explanation could be found in chromosome anomalies that affect boys. So far, the best known examples of these are cases with an extra X chromosome, which seems to cause a large number of learning problems (see for example Annell et al., 1970).

In fact, dyslexia research is characterized by lack of clarity, as well as disagreements, and uncertainty on many of the main points. This is probably an important reason why genetic research on dyslexia has not led to a larger number of definite results. At the same time, this also explains why an increasing number of new researchers are attacking the problems as inspiring riddles and exciting challenges.

Recent results of research

In *linkage* studies during recent years, it has again been assumed that a definite gene can cause dyslexia. The so-called linkage method is generally based on investigations over several generations. The more often two traits or properties occur together over several generations, the closer together the relevant genes are placed. If the localisation of one gene is known, the localisation of the other can be found. Smith et al. (1983) were the first to try linkage analyses in families with dyslexia over three generations. They considered that inheritance could be attributed to a gene on chromosome 15. More recently, there have been several investigations where linkage analysis has been used to study dyslexia (DeFries et al., 1991; Lubs et al., 1993; Smith et al., 1991). In addition to chromosome 15, attention has focused on chromosomes 1 and 6 (Cardon et al., 1994). In a linkage study, Grigorenko (1997) showed that defects of chromosomes 6 and 1 can give a deficit in phonological awareness, while word reading seems to be connected with chromosome 15. In order to determine more exactly where the genes are placed on the chromosome, more extensive and time-consuming work is needed (for an overview, see Rice, 1996).

The fact that we are well on the way to identifying the critical localisation of a possible dyslexia gene opens up both fascinating and frightening perspectives. If one succeeds in determining more exactly which genes are involved, an intensive study will begin on the manner in which genes take part in the synthesis of amino acids and in the construction of the nervous system. This can give us an unbelievably exciting insight into how the human body functions.

The second advantage of genetic knowledge is early diagnosis. In principle, a single test early in fetal life should show whether the fetus has a gene for dyslexia. It is easy to imagine the ethical problems that this raises.

Early identification could also lead to possible manipulation of the genome where the mutated genes could be exchanged for normal genes. This is still science fiction, but development is taking place very rapidly. The ethical discussion forces us to realize, even more strongly than before, that dyslexia is a deviation that cannot be compared with a well-defined somatic disease.

Brief Summary

Research on the biological causes of dyslexia is reductionistic in character, that is to say, attempts are made to discover the fundamental reasons why some people have such great problems with the written language. Neurological deviations have been found in dyslexics, but so far there are no diagnostic methods that can be used individually. In deceased dyslexics, small collections of brain cells, ectopias, have been found in the outer layer of the brain tissue. In the thalamus region, it has also been found that the magnocells for the visual system are smaller than normal, and that the cells in the relay station for hearing are also smaller than in normal readers. It is thought that this could be the cause of the dyslexic's difficulties with rapid perceptual events in both vision and hearing. However, some believe that this has nothing to do with writing difficulties in themselves, but merely reflects a general lag in the development of the nervous system.

We have also seen how, with new techniques, it is possible to study the brain in action in individuals with dyslexia. Compared with normal readers, dyslexics seem to process information in a different way when confronted with phonological tasks. The well-coordinated interaction between different areas of the brain that characterizes normal readers seems to be blocked in dyslexics.

Advances in genetics have also been used to look for the causes of dyslexia. In the first place, family and twin studies have shown that there is a strong hereditary element. However, the exact genetic course has been difficult to determine. It seems highly likely that dyslexia is influenced by many genes, which makes the question extra complicated. However, linkage analyses have shown that there are critical gene localisations on chromosomes 1, 6, and 15. However, we are still far from knowing more exactly which gene(s) is(are) involved, and which functions these genes then might have. Long before we have acquired this information, we must have an extensive ethical discussion on the consequences of the new knowledge.

CHAPTER 7

ASSESSMENT AND DIAGNOSING

A traditional view of teaching is that the teacher possesses knowledge which the pupil lacks, and the question is how to transfer or convey this knowledge to the pupil in the best possible way. This concept of conveyance of information in relation to teaching and knowledge is becoming increasingly out-of-date and misleading. An increasing number of researchers consider learning and the creation of knowledge as social processes where teachers and pupils enter into a partnership in which they jointly develop and construct understanding, ideas, and meaning. Parallel to the change in the way we look at knowledge, we have also seen a change in how pupils are regarded. The pupil is considered to be an active co-producer of meaning, and not a passive recipient of the teacher's organized signals. The pupil and the teacher have a communicative relationship to each other characterized by mutuality and respect.

It is important to have this perspective clearly in mind in a discussion about diagnosing. According to the traditional view, the teacher or the psychologist has several test instruments at his disposal. The pupil is assumed to adapt completely to the test leader. The instructions should be strictly followed, time limits adhered to, etc. When the diagnostic work is completed, the results are compared with a profile which ideally provides teachers and parents with guidance in the subsequent treatment. However, the diagnosis frequently only concludes with a label, which may be a relief, but which does not always provide constructive advice for remediation.

If teacher and pupil enter into an authentic communicative relationship, the diagnostic work must be given another character and direction. Perhaps the alternative strategy can best be illustrated by how we typically work with adult individuals with reading and writing disabilities. It is pretty obvious here that the adult will be expected to talk about the problems and the consequences they have had in his life. He will also often have hypotheses about the nature of the problems. After this, the conversation between the teacher/psychologist and the adult will form a basis for thoughts and ideas about relevant tests which can verify the hypothesis and throw new light on the problems. We are faced throughout with a problem-solving process where the tests only come in as a supporting element. In other words, we are not talking about following a test programme scrupulously or ritually, but rather a mutual investigation and assessment.

The diagnostic methods under consideration in this chapter should be examined on the basis of the approach to learning and pupils which we have touched on here. We will revert to other aspects of these important questions later, in the chapter on remediation.

The purpose of using tests can be found at several levels. Educational tests can be used in order to make a general assessment of knowledge and skills at a national level, which can in turn be used as a basis for political decisions regarding resource allocations. Sometimes it may also be of interest to make international comparisons. The IEA-investigation of reading skill in 9-year and 14-year old children is an example of this (Elley, 1994). Here, an attempt has been made to explain the variations in reading skill by means of various background facts, for example home environment, school resources, and teaching. In such contexts, the results of the individual is of limited interest.

Another purpose of larger, general assessment tests is to provide basic data for resource allocations at the local level. It may be necessary to assess the extent of reading difficulties in a municipality, or to find out how the problems vary from class to class. Yet another purpose of these assessment tests may be to observe the development and investigate whether the remediation has been effective.

Finally, we have diagnostic tests at the individual level, the purpose of which is to assess the strong and weak sides of the individual, and to find out whether there are factors that prevent good development in reading. Here, the test results should not primarily be used to provide diagnostic categories, but rather to give the teacher guidance in teaching and an instrument to appraise the effect of the remediation.

Someone has said that 'there is nothing more practical than a good theory'. Without theory, the diagnostic work may become unsystematic and fumbling, an effort where all sorts of information is collected without anyone really knowing how to use it. A diagnosis, based on theory, however, is well structured and systematic. We know what we want, we realize when we ought to stop, or when we need to proceed.

The overview of symptoms and causal factors in dyslexia in Chapter 1 can be used as a general theoretical steering system for the diagnostic work. Thus, it seems natural to assess word decoding and spelling as a first, important step. Our word decoding model in Chapter 2 and the spelling model in Chapter 3 will supply more detailed instructions. The underlying phonological problems should also be assessed in this context.

In connection with the diagnostic work, one should also look closely at certain 'closely related' language functions which - directly or indirectly - can have a negative effect on reading and/or writing. As teachers, we have, of course, no means of making neurological diagnoses. Nor do these have any educational implications at present.

It is, however, important for the teacher to take into consideration a few *related symptoms*, such as lack of attention, impulsiveness, sequencing, etc. Some *chance symptoms* may also be obstacles, for example visual defects or impaired hearing.

It is also important to look more closely at some of the *secondary symptoms*. To what extent can poor reading comprehension be due to poor word decoding? How is the sentence comprehension? Does the pupil have a sufficient vocabulary? What kind of metacognitive problems are there? To what extent has the pupil's self-esteem been influenced by the dyslexia?

Some of these questions should be addressed with 'softer' methods, using clinical-educational experience in talks with pupil, parents, teachers, and perhaps the health services. Other questions will include more formal test procedures.

As a general principle, there is no one, single diagnostic schema which is appropriate for all pupils with dyslexia. Each pupil is unique and has his own, unique configuration of strong and weak qualities. Therefore we must approach each pupil with great flexibility and insight. This is the very basis of a professional attitude. Professionals can, however, find good support in the use of carefully prepared and thoroughly tested diagnostic instruments. We present some such instruments in this chapter.

An Approach Based on Process Analysis

In teaching, it is often maintained that one should see a person as an entity, a sociocultural totality where feeling, thought, and will are inextricably united. We, too, think that such a perspective is basic in all practical teaching. We must meet the children with respect for their integrity as complete, responsible people.

In science however, abstractions and analyses have always been ambitions, i.e. an attempt is made to cultivate one or several aspects of a phenomenon, and isolate and investigate them, without disturbing the totality. Science and medicine have made great progress on the basis of this type of analytical strategy. But even in humanistic disciplines and sociology, there are examples of these analytical procedures being used, with progression from totality to the elements and subsequently back to totality.

Sometimes it is said that the whole is always more than the parts. For example, water is more than the sum of the components it is made from. Compared with its components, the properties of the water are *emergent*, i.e. new and not directly derivable from its separate parts. But even so, this emergence has not prevented chemists from using an analytical strategy in their research.

Ever since psychology emerged as a science a hundred years ago, an analytical strategy has been tried. As we are now attempting to gain more insight into the psychology of reading, we feel that analytical strategy should also be tried, even though we know that reading is an active, creative, constructive process. The question is whether we can gain anything by analyzing reading in more basic components. Such an attempt may turn out to be fruitful, at least in a dyslexia perspective.

We have seen that the primary problems of dyslexics can be localized to word decoding. All we have done here is to make an analytical distinction. Empirical experience can legitimize the distinction between decoding and comprehension. For example, most of us know how one can read aloud for children and not have the slightest idea of the content of what one has read. The decoding has clearly functioned on a highly automated level, while text comprehension has been totally disconnected, and thinking has proceeded in a quite different direction.

Now we take the analysis another step further to see whether the word decoding is divisible into components. The purpose of such analysis would be to acquire a theoretical understanding of the cognitive-linguistic architecture hidden behind the word decoding, i.e. the processes or components that enable us to recognize or write the word. If we get to know more about these processes, we may also have a chance to understand better at which points problems may arise for a dyslexic. Further elaboration of componential view of diagnosing reading difficulties is presented in volume edited by Joshi and Leong (1993).

We will call our attempts to understand what happens in word decoding *process analysis*. Such a strategy is different from what is sometimes called *functional analysis*. In functional analysis, reading *behaviour* is in focus. What can be observed during reading is described as well as possible, and above all the types of reading mistakes *The reading function is in focus*. The functional analytical strategy is reminiscent of the behaviourists' precise assessment of behaviour, where speculations about the underlying processes were scrupulously avoided because they could not be observed directly. On the basis of the functional description of reading and writing, advocates of functional analysis (for example, Gjessing, 1977), maintain that the observed symptoms can be placed in certain categories depending on the extent to which they indicate problems with the visual modality (sensory canal), or problems with the auditory modality. In a third category, we find symptoms where functions in both modalities have been disturbed.

By adopting modality thinking in functional analysis, one has in fact taken a step in the direction of process analysis, i.e. started to think of which processes lie behind the symptoms. However, in process analysis, this analysis is taken further.

Our object is to develop a model which describes the various steps in information processing when reading words. We stress that this is a model and not reality, in the same way as a diagram of London's Underground is not a picture of the actual tracks. Even so, the diagram gives the passengers a good idea of how the underground system functions.

So we outline a map or diagram of the cognitive-linguistic architecture of word decoding. This description of how a functioning system then forms the basis for understanding why dyslexics can have problems with decoding. The model provides guidance on the diagnostic strategy and makes it possible to discover which process or processes are not functioning satisfactorily.

One critical question then arises: Whether a model of a well-functioning system really can show how a disturbed or poorly developed system functions? In adults who have had their reading function disturbed because of brain damage, it may be easier to understand when limited or localized damage only affects one component of the total cognitive-linguistic architecture of word decoding. In such cases, we are talking about a well-functioning system built up through protracted training. The neuropsychological research literature on alexia, i.e. acquired dyslexia, strongly supports a process-analytical model where specific components can be injured, while other components function adequately.

But children with substantial decoding problems have not developed a functioning word decoding system. The following question should therefore be asked: Are not all the components of processing information so closely related that analytically separating them is impossible? In part, this is an empirical question which must be further investigated before a definite answer can be given. However, based on the experiences we have already made, we can maintain that dyslexics seem to have specific difficulties with phonological subprocesses. This prevents them from building well-functioning orthographic representations. Some dyslexics find it particularly difficult to recognize words directly, and have to use time-consuming and laborious sounding-out strategies in order to read the word.

Process analysis can be further developed, so that an even more exact clarification of which processes function poorly, and which function well, becomes possible. The object of this method of diagnosing is to clarify the individual processes. In order for process analysis to succeed, one needs a measuring instrument which measures the output from one component while the other components in the system are kept constant. Thus some components, which are suspected of having a direct influence on the process in question, are manipulated, and no others. If this strategy is successful, we have supportive evidence that the process-analytical model functions. If it turns out that all steps in the process are interdependent and interacting with each other all the time, it will be impossible to isolate the individual process, and the model can therefore not be tested.

An important aspect of a process-analytical model is therefore that we get ideas of how to proceed with the diagnostic process. As we shall see later, it may be relevant to measure reaction times and to expose the system to extreme load tests, for example short-term exposures. We will now see how process analysis can be used to clarify word decoding problems (see also Høien and Legaard, 1991).

Assessment of Word Decoding Problems

The purpose of assessment is to investigate which strategy or strategies the reader employs for decoding individual words, and to find out possible reasons why one or more strategies are not functioning.

Strategies in decoding single words

Here, the reader is asked to read several single words. The test leader records the number of correctly read words and makes a note of the reading errors, which will subsequently be given a qualitative analysis. The test leader also investigates whether the reader understands the words he reads, and records the number of words correctly understood. The response time will say something about the strategy employed. A short response time indicates that the orthographic strategy is being used, while a long response time indicates that the reader is using the more time-consuming phonological strategy.

An investigation of which linguistic dimensions of the word influence the decoding result, gives useful information on which strategy or strategies the reader uses during word decoding. Already at the stage where we see which words a reader finds difficult to decode, we know much about which decoding strategy the reader has used. However, one should be aware that most readers employ several strategies during word decoding, depending on the kind of word he is faced with.

Research has shown that there are at least eight linguistic dimensions of a word which have consequences for the use of strategy:

a) length of word
b) word/nonword
c) regularity/irregularity
d) abstract/concrete
e) content word/function word
f) homophone/non-homophone
g) frequency
h) phonological complexity

(a) The word length dimension
To some readers, it means a lot to the decoding result whether the word is long or short. In most cases, *long* words are difficult to read, but some readers have more trouble with some of the short words. When the reader has relatively more trouble with long words, it indicates that he uses the phonological strategy.

(b) The word/nonword dimension
Some readers have relatively greater difficulty in reading nonwords compared with their skill in reading real words. This indicates that they use the orthographic (or occasionally the logographic) strategy during word decoding, and that they find it difficult to use the phonological strategy, a strategy which must be intact if the nonwords are to be decoded correctly.

(c) The regularity/irregularity dimension
Regular words are the words that are pronounced in accordance with the most basic rules for grapheme-phoneme correspondence. Irregular words are those that will not be read correctly if the starting point is the usual grapheme-phoneme rules. The irregular words are only decoded correctly if the reader uses the orthographic strategy. When a reader has more difficulties with reading irregular than regular words, it indicates that he is using the phonological strategy in word decoding.

(d) The abstract/concrete dimension
In some readers, there is a dissociation in skills depending on the concrete/abstract dimension of the stimulus. A dissociation of this type indicates that the reader supports decoding with semantic cues. This happens most often when the orthographic strategy is used in word decoding. When using the phonological strategy, it is less important whether the stimulus word is concrete or abstract.

(e) Content word/function word dimension
Words can be classified in two main groups: content words and function words. The first group contains all the meaningful words and expressions. The function words

are those that bind the content words together syntactically. In some readers, we find a dissociation in skills dependent on whether the word is a content word or a function word. Some readers find it easier to read content words than function words. This dissociation indicates that the reader depends on semantic support in word decoding. When a pure phonological strategy is being used, it does not matter very much which word-class the stimulus words belongs to - provided that the other linguistic dimensions of the words are similar.

(f) The homophone/non-homophone dimension
Some readers experience problems when decoding words that are pronounced in the same way, but written differently (homophone words). Homophone words are orthographically different, and have a quite different semantic identity, but they all have the same phonological identity, i.e. they are pronounced the same way. One example of homophone words is *need* and *knead*. When the reader uses the orthographic strategy, he can easily retrieve the correct semantic identity parallel to the activating of the phonological identity. When he uses the phonological strategy, he is also able to read the word correctly, but he is uncertain when asked its meaning. It is essential that the reader knows that *kn* is pronounced /n/.

(g) The frequency dimension
Readers who use the orthographic strategy have a dissociation in skills, dependent on whether the stimulus word is met frequently or infrequently. The frequent words are those most often met by the reader during the reading process, and they are therefore easily recognized when encountered later on. The infrequent words are those that the reader rarely meets in normal texts, and it is thus not certain to what extent they have acquired orthographic identities in the long-term memory.

(h) The phonological complexity dimension
A stimulus word may have a complex or simple phonological structure. Phonologically complex words are words with consonant clusters, for example, *shrimp, fresh*. Simple phonological words are those that do not contain difficult and/or many consonants, for example, *sun, bell*. When the reader uses the orthographic strategy, it matters less whether the stimulus word is phonologically complex or simple. On the other hand, one finds a typical dissociation in decoding skill when the reader uses the phonological strategy.

We have now described how one can assess which decoding strategy the reader chooses to use when decoding words. In the next section, we will see how one can reduce the scope for choosing, and study the efficacy of the strategy that the reader has been forced to adopt.

Assessment of strategy skill

In order to find out whether a strategy functions satisfactorily, the test situation should ideally be arranged so that the reader can *only* use *this* strategy when decoding the word. In practice, however, this is not so simple.

Assessment of the orthographic strategy

Various tests have been designed to assess the orthographic strategy: Reading rapidly presented words (Høien and Lundberg, 1989a), reading irregular words (Coltheart, 1982), choosing between real words and homophonic nonwords (Olson et al., 1994), choosing between homophonic real words (Manis et al., 1990) and recognizing orthographic patterns (Vellutino, Scanlon and Tanzman, 1994). In all tests, both the number of correct answers and reaction time are registered. The reaction time is the time from the presenting of the word until the answer is given. By using a computer with microphone one gets a very exact measurement of the reaction time.

1. Reading quickly presented words
In tachistoscopic presentation of a word, the stimulus time is very short, for example a fraction of a second. It is therefore difficult for the reader to obtain a good result if he uses the phonological strategy. The result of word decoding will depend largely on how well the reader masters the orthographic strategy. Reading of tachistoscopically presented words can therefore provide information on the reader's orthographic skills.

2. Reading irregular words
As we noted in Chapter 3, most words are neither regular nor irregular, but something in between. That is, 'regularity' comes in varying degrees. The words we usually call 'irregular' are those whose spelling rules are somewhat uncommon, for example *rough* and *wrong*. Neither of these are *totally* irregular: after all, the *-ough* spelling (and the 'uff' sound) is used in a lot of words, as is the silent *w* in *wrong*. Some irregular words, however, don't follow any rules, such as *people, have, of,* and a few others. They are cases unto themselves. In accordance with the traditional dual-route model, irregular words cannot be decoded by means of the phonological strategy. However, irregular words can be decoded by means of the orthographic strategy. If, in addition to this, the irregular words are presented with a short exposure time, even greater demands are made on efficient orthographic processing to obtain an adequate result.

3. Choosing between real words and homophonic nonwords
This test consists of ordinary words and nonwords whose spelling yields the same pronunciation as the real word. Examples would be *car* and *kar*, or *played* and *plade*. If the reader employs the phonological strategy, without back-up help from an orthographic recognition process, there is no way that he can distinguish the word from its homophonic nonword. The only way to solve this kind of problem is to use the orthographic strategy.

4. Choosing between homophones
In this test, a sentence is read to the pupil, and then two homophonic real words are presented. Only one of them fits the context. An example: 'I need a pen'. Then, *need* and *knead* are presented, and the pupil is asked to mark the one that fits. A correct

answer depends on orthographic skill, since the pronunciation of the words is identical, and thereby, yields no help for making a correct choice.

5. Recognizing orthographic patterns

This is a relatively new test concept which has proved to be an efficient assessment of orthographic knowledge (Siegel, Geva and Share, 1992). The pupil is presented with two nonwords, and is asked to decide which of them looks most like a word. Examples would be *braflge-blage, orabg-orbag, caog-cogl*. Both nonwords can be read off by means of the phonological strategy - if you really try. But only one of the pair conforms to fairly common spelling rules. In each of the examples, the first member of each pair breaks fairly clearly with the orthotactical rules of English (see Chapter 3) - which is why it looks weird - while the second member conforms to fairly common rules. Even though they can be pronounced, the phonological strategy does not help the child to discover which of the nonwords *looks most like* a word. In order to answer that question, a child needs to have a 'feel' for spelling, that is, a sensitivity to orthographic structures.

Assessment of the phonological strategy

Various tests have been used to assess the phonological strategy: Reading nonwords aloud, choosing which of nonwords in accordance with a read nonword, and choosing nonwords which are homophone to a real word (Olson et al., 1994).

1. Reading nonwords

When investigating the reader's skill in using the phonological strategy, one must ensure that the test situation is arranged so that other strategies are excluded as far as possible. This is the case when the task is to read a completely unknown regular word. It is, however, difficult to make quite certain that the stimulus word is one hundred per cent unknown to the reader, and thus it is not completely possible to exclude use of the orthographic strategy. On the other hand, if one uses nonwords as stimulus words (for example *biba, klast, jinen, sabin,* etc.), one knows that they are not represented by orthographic identities in dictionaries, and we can assume that the decoding result will depend largely on the functional level of the phonological strategy. However, orthographic knowledge can also be used to read nonwords, if they look like real words orthographically. Therefore, it is very important that the nonwords are as orthographically different from real words as possible.

2. Choosing nonwords that are homophone to read nonwords

In this test, a nonword (for example *metoso*) is read aloud to the pupil. The pupil repeats the nonword to ensure that it has been perceived correctly. The pupil is then presented with two written nonwords, and is asked to choose the one with the spelling that corresponds to the word that has been read.

3. Choosing a homophone nonword

This test can be used to measure the phonological strategy. The pupil is presented with several nonwords. The pronunciation of half the nonwords is like that of a real word. The task is to mark these nonwords. There are different ways of presenting the nonwords. Some have chosen to present them in pairs, i.e. with a homophone nonword (for example *rong*) and a non-homophone nonword (*jong*). Others have chosen to present the nonwords one by one in an arbitrary order. The task is to choose the nonwords that sound like real words.

Analysis of errors

When strategy skills are being assessed, an analysis of the errors made during the word decoding test is also carried out. The error analysis includes categorization of the reading errors in certain error categories. Through an analysis of the reading errors, information is obtained that can be used when evaluating strategy use and skills. However, it is not easy to carry out an analysis of this kind, and it is even more complicated to interpret the result of the analysis reliably. This should be kept in mind when discussing the various error categories.

The most frequently categories are these:

> a) visual defects
> b) phonological errors
> c) semantic errors
> d) derivation errors
> e) function word replacements
> f) regularisation errors
> g) neologisms
> h) omissions and additions of letters

(a) Visual errors
Visual errors occur where the response word (the answer) is visually related to the stimulus word, for example *him-his*. This type of error is frequently found when readers use the orthographic strategy, but the errors show that the strategy is not working satisfactorily.

(b) Phonological errors
Phonological errors are faulty readings where the sound of the response word is related to the stimulus word, for example *ball-pall*. This type of error often appears when the phonological strategy is used, and the misreading shows that the strategy is not working adequately.

(c) Semantic errors
Here, the reading error occurs where the meaning of the response word is related to the stimulus word, for example *she-woman, gift-present, soul-angel.*

(d) Derivation errors
Some readers have a tendency to omit or add word suffixes, for example *sunny* is read as *sun*, *bench* as *benches*, *lovely* as *love*, etc. These reading mistakes are called derivation errors, and they occur particularly often when using the orthographic

strategy. The errors indicate that the strategy is not functioning properly.

(e) Function word replacements
Sometimes the response word is a completely different word from the stimulus word. This happens most frequently when function words are read. For example, The word *under* is read as *on, and* becomes *or*, etc. Thus, the stimulus word is replaced by an other function word meaning something quite different, and the response word has no likeness to the stimulus word, visually or phonologically. Function word replacements occur in particular when the reader employs the orthographic strategy, and indicate that this strategy is not functioning properly.

(f) Regularizations
These are reading errors where the response word is read out directly in accordance with the most common rules for grapheme-phoneme correspondence, for example, when the word *island* is read as /is/*land* instead of /i/*land*. These errors are associated with the use of the phonological strategy. If irregular words are to be read correctly, the reader must use the orthographic strategy or have adopted linguistic memory aids (for example, '*You* is spelled /y/o/u/'.

(g) Neologisms
Sometimes, a word is decoded as a nonword, for example, *shake* turns into *hakey*, *rarely* into *sairly*, etc. These errors are called neologistic errors, and they show that the reader uses the phonological strategy when decoding the stimulus word. The errors show that this strategy does not function properly.

(h) Omissions and adding of letters
We often find that one or several letters are omitted from or added to the word. This type of error occurs particularly in connection with the use of the phonological strategy, but the errors show that the strategy does not function satisfactorily.

So far, we have remained on a basic and fundamental level when discussing how to organize the diagnostic strategy when assessing word decoding. In the next section, we will give an example of a computer-based diagnostic programme, which is built on the principles we have outlined (Høien and Lundberg, 1989b).

KOAS

'KOAS' is a *word decoding test.* (In Norwegian KOAS is an abbreviation for Assessment of Word Decoding Strategies.) It is different from other diagnostic reading tests in that it builds directly on a theory regarding word decoding (Høien and Lundberg, 1989a, b). By means of 'KOAS', the decoding strategies used when reading single words are assessed.

The word lists in 'KOAS' are made in such a way that they give as exact information as possible on the reader's choice of strategy and strategy skill when reading single words and nonwords. By systematically varying the linguistic factors that are thought to affect the decoding process, their effect on the answer given is measured. This knowledge gives insight into how the decoding strategies function.

KOAS assesses the decoding strategies by means of five different tests (see Figure 2.2 in Chapter 2):

Assessing the use of strategy:
1. Reading words aloud with a long time limit (test 1.1)

Assessing the orthographic strategy:
2. Reading words aloud with a short time limit (test 2.1)
3. Distinguishing between words that can be pronounced the same way. (test 2.2)

Assessing the phonological strategy:
4. Reading nonwords aloud(test 3.1)
5. Distinguishing between nonwords and homophone nonwords (test 3.2)

In order to find out whether a strategy functions satisfactorily, the various subtests (with the exception of test 1) are made in such a way that the reader is forced to use a certain strategy when decoding words.

In test 1.1, the test subject can choose the reading strategy freely. In test 2.1, the words are presented tachistoscopically. In this way, the possibility of obtaining a satisfactory result with the phonological strategy is very limited. Test 2.2 gives additional information on the reader's skill in using the orthographic strategy, but this time without the time limitation. Test 2.2 also excludes the use of a possible logographic strategy, since the reader can solve these problems correctly only if he has established well-specified orthographic identities. In test 3.1, the phonological strategy is assessed. The nonwords are read aloud, and one should be aware that articulatory difficulties may have a negative effect on the test result. Test 3.2 gives more information on how effective the phonological strategy is functioning. This test does not make any demands on the articulation of the words, but on phonological word recognition.

In the evaluation of the results, all available information should be included: the number of correct answers, response time for correctly read words and nonwords, how the linguistic dimensions of the word influences the decoding result, the result of the error analysis, as well as the response time for words and nonwords not read correctly. In addition, the test leader has also collected information on the reading behaviour of the test subject: Does he use letter reading or sounding out? Does he split the words into syllables? How is the articulation and the intonation?

The next natural step in our process-analytical diagnosis programme will be to assess the individual processes behind the decoding strategies.

Assessment of word decoding processes

We realize that it is difficult to find tests that only assess one process. Even in the simplest tests, several processes are frequently involved. We must keep this in mind when the results are assessed. The tests that we refer to below were used when diagnosing the test subjects and control pupils in the Dyslexia Project in Stavanger (Høien and Lundberg, 1989c). We chose to call this test the KOAP test (In Norwegian KOAP is an abbreviation for Assessment of Word Decoding Processes.) The following subprocesses were used (see Figure 2.2 in Chapter 2):

a) assessment of the visual perception process
b) assessment of letter identification
c) assessment of the word recognition process
d) assessment of the phonological recollection process
e) assessment of the semantic activating process
f) assessment of the parsing process
g) assessment of the phonological recoding process
h) assessment of the phonological synthesis

The correct score and the reaction time were converted to a value that was used as an aggregate measure of the pupil's skill in mastering the individual strategy. Based on these results, one could draw the process profile of each individual pupil, showing his weak and strong skills. All pupils who took part in the Dyslexia Project in Stavanger were tested using KOAS and KOAP.

Even though all the dyslexics except one showed a poor skill in the phonological strategy, i.e. nonword reading, the process profile varied from pupil to pupil. This was even more evident when we included in the test battery the tests of the pupils' verbal short-term memory and their skill in phonological analysis. This goes to show that poor skill in using one decoding strategy may be due to a failure of various decoding processes.

The process analysis also shows that the dyslexics have managed to compensate for their phonological difficulties to a varying extent. It was also interesting to see how the same process profile was in fact present in those of the parents who had reading difficulties (Høien et al., 1989).

The dyslexics did not deviate from the control pupils in respect of visual or semantic processes. On the other hand, when tested in phonological synthesis skill, their score was particularly poor. In some tasks, for example assessing phonological recoding of letters, the dyslexics had a longer reaction time than the control pupils. We found that the measurement of reaction time is very important when gaining insight in how automated a decoding process is.

The Dyslexia Research Foundation has recently developed and standardized a new version of the KOAP-test which assesses exactly the various sub-components assumed to be involved in early reading acquisition (Oftedal and Høien, 1997). This test is also based on the theoretical model for word decoding which has been explained in this book (see Chapter 2).

Word Chain Test

The test *Word chain* was first produced in 1987. It was part of a large test battery in the multidisciplinary research project 'Leseutvikling i Kronoberg' (Reading development in Kronoberg) in Sweden. An English version of the Word chain test is now available (Miller Guron, 1999).

The word chain test is a short and simple group test which can be used to assess decoding skill and word recognition. It can also be used as an individual test. It only takes about 15 minutes to perform the test in a whole class, including instruction time. The tasks consist of indicating by a pencil stroke where there should be a space between words in a sequence consisting of four words written consecutively. In the course of 4 minutes the pupils are asked to mark as many *word* boundaries as possible. The test contains 90 word chains such as: *wordarrowwoodwho, treeoverlifesee, soursmallerfreecow*, etc.

The length of the words in the test varies between two and seven letters. The words are nouns, verbs, adjectives, adverbs, prepositions, and names of digits. The test is simple and easy to correct.

The word chain test can be used to gain an idea of the pupil's technical reading skill. The test can also be used as a screening test to discover pupils with reading problems. It may also be relevant to use the word chain test as an individual test to assess how far a child or an adult (for example in adult education) has progressed in the development of word decoding.

Assessment of Reading Text Aloud

It is also important to assess how the dyslexic reads texts aloud. By using texts of varying degrees of difficulty, it is possible to investigate whether the degree of difficulty affects the pupil's way of reading, the speed of reading, and reading comprehension.

While the text is being read, one should also take note of the reading behaviour: Does the pupil use sounding out or letter reading? Are there frequent pauses, hesitations, and guesses on the basis of the context? What is the intonation like? This type of information is important when assessing decoding skill. One can investigate to what extent the pupil makes use of the context to support word decoding by comparing the skill in decoding single words with reading consecutive text.

Assessment of Spelling

Different types of tasks can be used to assess spelling skill. The most common are dictation of words, writing nonwords, dictation of sentences, and free compositions. The degree of difficulty of the tests must naturally be related to the age and skill level of the pupil.

An analysis of spelling mistakes made by the dyslexic provides useful information on which strategy or strategies he uses when spelling words, and how well these strategies function. Specially designed tasks also make it possible to gain more insight into the separate processes behind the spelling strategies.

Which words are difficult to spell correctly?

As with word decoding, we find that different dimensions of the word affect spelling differently depending on the spelling strategy used by the dyslexic. When we see which word dimensions create difficulties in spelling, we know something about which strategy has been used and how well that strategy functions. The following word dimensions are of special interest: word length, degree of phonological complexity, and whether the word is regular or not.

If the error frequency increases in proportion to the length of the word, this indicates that the dyslexic is using a phonological strategy. The more sounds you have to encode the greater the change of making a mistake. If spelling mistakes are found particularly in phonologically complex words, this indicates again that the spelling is using the phonological strategy. When the phonological strategy is used, there is also an obvious difference in the number of errors between regular and irregular words, with a clear accumulation of spelling mistakes of irregular words. A word is therefore irregular compared with the reader's alphabetic knowledge of phoneme-grapheme correspondence.

When a reliable orthographic strategy is used, there is no clear relationship between the number of errors and the degree of phonological complexity of the word, or the degree to which the word is regular or not. Moreover, the length of the word does not very much affect the result of the spelling either.

Analysis of spelling mistakes

The assessment must also include an analysis of the spelling mistakes made by the dyslexic (see also chapter 4). Here, it is important to find out whether certain letters or sounds are confused, whether letters are omitted or added to the word, and whether capital and small letters are used correctly. When a text is written, one can see whether, for example, two words are joined together as one word, whether a single word is divided into two *words* (a bout for about*)*, and whether punctuation marks are used correctly. Deficiencies in these fields probably reflect a defective metasyntactic and morphological awareness, and a general linguistic weakness. Naturally, the greatly reduced experience of reading and writing will contribute to these types of spelling mistakes.

When assessing spelling, one must naturally also remember factors such as the amount of emphasis put on spelling in the lessons, the age of the pupil, and his dialect. Many spelling mistakes that are first interpreted as phonological confusions are in fact due to dialect. Spelling mistakes like this do not indicate phonological deficiencies, but on the contrary that the pupil functions well phonologically. The pupil writes the sounds correctly based on his articulation of the words, and his knowledge of fundamental letter-sound associations.

Research has not been able to demonstrate that dyslexics make different qualitative spelling mistakes from other pupils. It is more a question of the number of mistakes than the type of mistake. It is characteristic of dyslexics that they have so many spelling mistakes, and that the mistakes tend to persist even if the reading difficulties disappear. They add to and omit letters from words, confuse phonemes that sound similar, and they frequently regularize even highly frequent words.

Assessment of Written Work

The diagnostic process should not be limited to an analysis of the pupil's spelling mistakes. Written work produced by the pupil is an important element of the diagnostic process, enabling us to carry out an extended analysis including factors such as clearness of presentation, progression, relevance, and personal style.

Santa (1995) points out six fields that are important when assessing written work: *Content, organization, personal style, choice of words, sentences,* and *conventions.* Below follows a brief description of each of these:

1. Content
Strength
>Keeps to the main theme
>Clear details and examples
>Knows the theme, writes from experience

Weakness
>Jumps from one topic to another
>Lack of details
>Not credible

2. Organization
Strength
>The introduction makes one want to read more
>The composition has a natural framework
>The details support the main theme
>The story has a natural end

Weakness
>No introduction
>Difficult to see order in the presentation
>The main theme is poorly substantiated
>No end or conclusion

3. Personal style
Strength
>Presentation *vivid* and with a personal style

Weakness
>Other people's thoughts and ideas
>Lifeless

4. Choice of words
Strength
>Vivid description
>Varied vocabulary

Relevant concepts
Weakness
Unimaginative use of words
Lacks relevant concepts

5. Sentences
Strength
Complete sentences
Sentences vary in both length and structure
Easy to read aloud
Weakness
Incomplete sentences
Same pattern of sentences is repeated

6. Conventions
Strength
Correct spelling
Correct punctuation
Correct conjugations
Correct layout as regards paragraphs, etc.
Weakness
Many spelling mistakes
Many punctuation mistakes
Many conjugation mistakes
No division into natural paragraphs

As the instruction in writing progresses, the effect of the instruction should be assessed continuously. The main object of the assessment is to ensure that the pupil, teacher, and parents are all informed of the child's progress. Meaningful assessment takes into account the situation in which teaching and learning are taking place.

The assessment is meant to help the pupils to see what they have learnt, and what they still find difficult to master. The assessment therefore provides a starting point for deciding which targets the individual pupil should aim at during the next period. Here, a *portfolio* is a useful tool. A portfolio is a selection of the pupil's written work. The pupil chooses which work should be included in the file. Each piece of written work is dated and filed separately, forming the basis for individual conversations and evaluation (Santa, 1995).

Assessment of Phonological Problems

Dyslexia is primarily a deficiency in the phonological field. This deficiency is particularly evident in tasks that demand phonological coding. The dyslexic therefore has difficulty in mastering several phonological sub-skills such as phoneme parsing and synthesis, letter-sound association, orthographic pattern-sound pattern association, naming letters and words, and verbal memorizing. A thorough assessment of phonological sub-skills should always be an important part of the diagnostic procedure in dyslexia.

1. Assessment of the phonological awareness

Phoneme parsing is one of the most frequently used tests in connection with the assessment of phonological awareness. A word is read to the pupil who has to repeat all the phonemes in the word in the right order. Another test that is used is phoneme deletion. The pupil is once again given a word and has to find out which word is left when the first sound is deleted (e.g. *bring* becomes *ring*).

Sometimes older pupils and adults find this type of task too simple. Then, an alternative is to use so-called spoonerism tasks. Research has shown that adult dyslexics have great difficulty in performing this type of task with a normal reaction time. In a spoonerism, two words are given, for example Pat Boon. The challenge is to switch the two first sounds and then state which new words have been formed. In our example the correct answer is Bat Poon. In addition to skill in phonemic analysis, spoonerism tasks also make demands on verbal memory.

2. Assessment of phoneme synthesis

When starting to learn to read, sound blending is essential in order to decode words. Research shows that skill in phoneme synthesis does not come automatically as a result of skill in phoneme parsing (Wagner, Torgesen and Rashotte, 1994). The two sub-skills differ in some ways, and both are important in connection with learning to read. It is therefore important to assess both in the diagnostic process.

3. Assessment of verbal short-term memory (V-STM)

Verbal short-term memory is important in learning to read, both as regards word decoding and reading comprehension. Poor verbal memory makes the synthesis process difficult, specially when it is built on single sounds. Sounding out gives the reader a starting point in a recoding of sound of each single letter in the word. The sounds are stored temporarily in the short-term memory, and this material then forms the basis for synthesis. If the short-term memory is poor, some of the sounds will disappear from the memory before the synthesis process can be carried out. The reader is in a particularly bad position if the letter-sound associations have not become automatic, which delays recoding and puts an even heavier load on the short-term memory. When assessing the verbal short-term memory it is therefore important to present the letter sounds auditively, not visually. Several other tests can also be used to assess verbal short-term memory. In some tests the test subject has to memorize and repeat a certain number of words or nonwords. Another variant is based on sentences. Two or three sentences are read aloud and the test subject is asked to state an opinion on an allegation in each sentence. Then he/she is asked to memorize the last word in each sentence.

When assessing verbal short-term memory, it is important to remember the negative effect that feelings, need for achievement, and concentration problems may have on the test result. One cannot therefore immediately conclude that a low score indicates poor verbal short-term memory. But if the reader has genuine difficulties with short-term memory, this must be taken into consideration when choosing which method of instruction should be used. A reading method based on larger orthographic units than individual letters, i.e. common letter combinations, will not make the same demands on the short-term memory capacity as a method based on single sounds.

4. Assessment of the ability to name objects rapidly

Research has shown that the ability to name drawings rapidly of known objects, colours, digits, and letters makes up a distinct phonological factor, separate from other phonological factors such as phonological awareness. According to Wolf and Segal (1992), pupils with a condition they describe as *double deficit* are in the worst position when learning to read: These pupils are those with the most serious reading problems because they are inadequate as regards phonological awareness and also have difficulty in naming objects.

Two tasks can be used to assess naming problems: 1) Naming drawings of known objects (from semantic identity to articulation), and 2) Naming letters. In both cases the stimuli are presented one at a time. An alternative method is to present five drawings in a random order and assess the number of objects correctly named in the course of a short period (e.g. 2 minutes). Instead of drawings of objects one can also use different colours, digits, or letters.

5. Assessment of ability to repeat words and nonwords

Dyslexics seem to have more difficulty than normal readers in repeating words and nonwords. This is most obvious with repetition of phonologically complicated nonwords (e.g. with unusual consonant clusters). One may ask what it is that causes the repetition problems. Several answers are possible: 1) poor phonological perception, 2) difficulty in activating phonological codes, 3) faulty connection between phonological and articulatory codes, 4) difficulties with performing articulation, or 5) poor short-term memory.

Assessment of Morphological Awareness

It can be said that writing uses two main principles to express language. The phonological principle, which we have focused on until now, is not sufficient. We want the origin and relationship of words to each other to appear in writing as well. We therefore have a morphological principle, which means that the words are spelt the same although the pronunciation changes with conjugations and derivations. For example we write *knee* but we say *nee*. The spelling is based on the morphological principle that aims at retaining the connection with the Old Norse *kne*.

It has been shown that many dyslexic children do not always understand or are conscious of the morphological structure of words. Elbro (1990) has investigated this thoroughly, and has also developed a number of tasks to be used when testing morphological awareness. For example, it is possible to compare reading words with and without semantic morpheme cues, for example *out*come-April, *car*s-hut, or words with or without a semantic morpheme cue at the beginning, for example *sun*dial-sledge, *re*search-thirst.

Assessment of Reading Comprehension

A test of reading comprehension usually contains a short text of 10-20 lines followed by questions on the content, usually as multiple choice. Sometimes a *cloze test* is used, i.e. every fifth or sixth word is removed and the pupil is asked to fill in the spaces. In order to succeed here, the pupil must be able to benefit from the context and understand the content.

There are also texts which only test the pupil's ability to understand single sentences. The pupil reads a sentence and is told to choose which of six pictures fits in best with the content of the sentence.

In reality, reading is seldom a question of thorough scrutiny of a series of consecutive sections of text. The conventional tests do not give a very good picture of how a child can actually perform under more natural reading conditions. Reading may consist of many different things, a rapid glance at a street sign, following a recipe, looking for a name in a catalogue, looking up a word in a dictionary, reading subtitles on television, following the course of events in a story, understanding the point of a story, interpreting the intentions of the author, criticizing his arguments, and assessing whether a text is appropriate. Strictly speaking, all these texts and types of task should be included when testing the reading skill of a pupil. This means that a good deal of work on the diagnosis has to take place informally in connection with daily routines in the classroom.

The diagnosis should also include an assessment of the child's previous knowledge in relation to the text used. Other important aspects to assess are the children's attitude to reading, and their reading habits. What do they usually read in their free time? How often? For how long? What is the purpose? Do they read because they want to or because they have to? What do they think of the different texts? Answers to this type of question can provide useful information in the attempt to foster a love of reading in the pupil, which is essential in order to progress with teaching.

Assessment of Metacognition

Assessment of the metacognitive strategy of the pupil is closely related to assessment of reading comprehension. Here there are almost no formal or informal tests or questionnaires available. You have to talk to the pupil and observe his behaviour in order to obtain a picture of how he works, and what his attitude is to reading, and how aware he is of what reading consists of.

By talking to the pupil, you get a feeling for the extent to which he is aware that it is possible to have different goals when reading, and that different goals may entail different ways of reading. Does the pupil always read in the same way and at the same speed regardless of the type of text, or does he try to adjust his reading to the text and the goal? Does he sometimes skim through the text and sometimes read more thoroughly? Does he underline or mark certain sections in factual texts? Does he notice if he makes a mistake when reading? Does he notice when he does not understand? Does he ask himself: 'What is this about?' Does he make summaries? Does he usually know whether what he is reading seems reasonable, credible? If he does not understand a text, what does he do? Does he read the whole text again or only parts of it? Does he keep at it to see if he can succeed? Does he ask questions? Does he give up and put the text aside? The list of questions can be continued. However, the main point is to see to which extent the pupil makes use of active strategies in order to read.

In Umeå, Sweden, a data technique has been developed (Jarvella et al., 1989) where only a portion of the text is visible on the screen at one time. The text can be read by following the window as it moves along the text line. The reader can regulate the speed of the window. This technique showed that poor readers always kept the same reading speed regardless of whether the text was difficult or easy. On the other hand, good readers adjusted the speed of reading according to how difficult it was and to the object of the reading. We deliberately introduced some mistakes into the text to see how quickly the readers noticed them. We told the readers in advance that there were mistakes in the text. The poor readers seldom noticed these mistakes, even though some of them made the content of the text completely incomprehensible. This type of data technique is not yet available for practical diagnosis, but we expect great future developments in this field.

We have now given an account of how we can assess the different aspects of reading and writing. In the last part of this chapter we will look at the different obstacles to the reading and writing process and see how they can be assessed.

Assessing Obstacles to Good Reading

As mentioned previously, there are a number of related and sporadic symptoms in those with reading problems which can obstruct the process of learning to read. When we use the word *obstacle* we indicate that the factor in question is a part of the poor readers' problem. However, it should be remembered that there is usually a complicated interaction going on. An obstructive factor may arise as a consequence of either an unsuccessful attempt at learning to read or lack of reading experience. In non-dyslexic pupils, these factors do not always have a negative effect on reading, but in the vulnerable dyslexics they may be the 'last straw', making a big problem even bigger. We will take a closer look at some of the commonest obstacles: poor intellectual ability, poor linguistic functions, visual defects, impaired hearing, emotional and motivational problems, poor stimulation in the home environment, and negative factors connected with education.

Poor intellectual ability

We have pointed out that there is not a strong correlation between intellectual ability and decoding skill. A minor degree of decreased intellectual ability is therefore not a serious obstacle to the technical side of learning to read. However, if the intellectual ability is further decreased, this will naturally have a negative effect on the pupil's ability to acquire an effective decoding skill quickly. This must have educational consequences for both the choice of method and the progression in teaching. Intellectual ability has a great effect on the comprehension process. Therefore, in order to avoid underachievement and defeat, it is important that teachers adjust the content, speed of instruction, and teaching method to the intellectual ability of the individual pupil.

Even in a pupil with normal intellectual ability, the cognitive profile may be very uneven. We often see pupils with poor verbal short-term memory and sequencing problems. A weakness in these cognitive areas will have a negative effect on the first attempts to learn to read.

Assessment of the intellectual level is often integrated into the routine dyslexia diagnostic procedure. We have pointed out that dyslexia can occur at all levels of intelligence, but if there is also poor intellectual ability, the reading and writing problems will naturally be even greater than otherwise. Poor intellectual ability has a particularly negative effect on the comprehension process.

When assessing cognitive resources, it is important not to use intelligence tests that make demands on reading and writing skills. This kind of test does not give a correct picture of the dyslexic's general cognitive resources. The performance sections of WISC-R and Raven's matrices are suitable for giving a correct picture of the general cognitive development in pupils with reading and writing problems.

We are not only interested in gaining knowledge of the pupil's general intellectual abilities. It is just as important, if not more important, to gain knowledge of the dyslexic's *cognitive profile*. The WISC-R test is well suited for assessing this. This test consists of a series of subtests that provide useful information on the ability to handle numbers, remember numbers, word comprehension, reasoning, and visuo-spatial skills.

Much research has been carried out on the use of WISC-R in diagnosing dyslexia (Searls, 1987). In general, dyslexics score less well in the verbal part of the test than in the performance part. Many studies also show that dyslexics have a special profile regarding the results of WISC-R, the so-called ACID profile. They score particularly poorly in arithmetic (A), coding (C), information (I), and short-term memory (digit span, D).

Delayed language development

Linguistic skills are important in order to be able to learn to read. By linguistic skills we mean comprehension of concepts, vocabulary, syntactic competence, and articulatory skill. Pupils with delayed language development therefore encounter special difficulties when learning to read. This obstructive mechanism has an especially marked effect on reading comprehension, but also has a negative effect on word decoding.

In a large investigation on 700 pupils in the first grade, Lundberg (1985) showed that the pupils' ability to comprehend and produce language is the most important factor for predicting progress in reading later at school. This is not surprising, since reading is primarily a linguistic function.

As mentioned previously, different types of linguistic difficulties (closely related symptoms) are found in connection with dyslexia. Assessment of language skill must therefore include concept comprehension, vocabulary, syntax, and articulation.

Visual deficits

The visual process is the first, introductory process behind reading. Reduced visual function will therefore have a negative effect on all the later processes that lead to word decoding.

The visual defects that may be connected with reading disabilities can affect the fields of *visual acuity, field of vision,* and *binocular vision.* If there is the slightest suspicion that a pupil's reading problems could be connected with visual defects, his or her vision must be investigated thoroughly. It should also be remembered that a minor visual defect may have a more negative effect in pupils with dyslexia than in pupils with normal reading abilities (for an overview, see Willows, Kruk and Corcos, 1993).

If it is suspected that there is something wrong with vision, the teacher should contact the school health services and ask for a thorough examination of vision. The teacher should also collect qualitative data by talking to the pupil about his/her problems. We should not forget that the pupil often has good insight and understanding of his/her own problems, and that this information is an important supplement to the more objective data that are collected in optometric examinations.

As mentioned previously, recent research has pointed out that if the after-image of a visual impression lasts too long (long iconic persistence), this can make the reading process more difficult because the sensory stimulus from one fixation masks the next sensory impression. There is a special apparatus that can measure iconic persistence, but it is expensive. A simple test is to see whether it is easier for a poor reader if a blue transparent sheet is placed over the text. In theory, this diminishes masking, while it is increased if a red transparent sheet is used.

Impaired hearing

Impaired hearing also obstructs learning to read. There may be a general loss of hearing affecting all the frequencies or a more specific loss of hearing, limited to one or more frequency zones.

The extent to which impaired hearing affects learning to read will depend on how much of the reading instruction is verbal. A loss of hearing prevents phonological word decoding because the pupil is not able to differentiate similar phonemes. Both the phonological analysis and synthesis therefore become problematic. The loss of hearing may also make learning of concepts difficult, and thus have a negative effect on the comprehension process.

Some investigations have also shown that poor readers may have subtle hearing problems that cannot be found with the traditional hearing tests (Høien, 1982). These problems depend partly on how long the sensory stimulus is available in the echoic memory, and partly on problems with processing rapid sequences of sound. A possible hypothesis, which has not been confirmed, is that these problems could be behind the dyslexic's phonological difficulties.

The apparatus used to test hearing is called an audiometer, and the results are recorded on an audiogram. In audiology, two units are often mentioned when sound is described: hertz (Hz) and decibel (dB). Hertz is a measure of the frequency number of sound waves per second. The human ear can usually hear sound waves from 16 Hz up to 20,000 Hz. Speech sounds are mostly in the region 500-6000 Hz, and vowel sounds have a lower frequency than most consonant sounds. A hearing loss can therefore affect the learning of different language sounds, depending on which frequency is impaired. It is therefore important that special teachers know the hearing curve of the pupils so that they can compare these with the knowledge of which frequency zones are most critical for each language sound.

Decibel is the unit of volume- the level of sound pressure compared to the sound that can just be heard by those with normal hearing: the normal lower limit is 0 dB. It is not considered that variations between 0-15 dB affect auditive perception. However, a hearing loss of over 15 dB may have a negative effect on the perception process.

Emotional and motivational problems

It is extremely difficult to see what is cause and what is effect in the relationship between emotional and motivational problems and poor reading skill.

Can dyslexia lead to social and emotional problems, or is it the social and emotional problems that make it difficult to learn to read and write? Which comes first, the chicken or the egg? There are no unambiguous data that can answer this question. However, there is one investigation that approaches the problem. Pennington et al. (1993) studied three groups of pupils. One group had purely dyslexic symptoms without having emotional problems. They were well-adjusted and fairly quiet pupils who fought their battle with letters without making a fuss. Another group was characterized as ADHD (attention deficit with hyperactivity disorder). They had great difficulties with concentration. They could not sit still and were restless and noisy in the classroom. On the plus side, they did not have special difficulties with reading and writing. A third group had both ADHD symptoms and difficulties with both reading and writing.

The groups were tested in two ways. There were phonological tests (e.g. reading nonwords, rhyme tasks, secret language as Pig-Latin type exercises, phoneme parsing), and tests that measured concentration and the ability to persevere, attend, and be accurate. Not unexpectedly, the purely dyslexic group managed the phonological tasks poorly, but managed well in the executive tasks. The opposite was found in the ADHD group. The crucial question was how the mixed group fared. It turned out that they had the same pattern as the purely dyslexic group.

A reasonable interpretation of this result is that the mixed group had developed their socioemotional problems as a consequence of the problems associated with dyslexia. Lack of concentration, noisiness, and aggression were clearly not *true* ADHD problems associated with disturbances in brain function. Before drawing too definite conclusions on cause and effect here, one should await more investigations of the same kind, preferably designed so that they follow the pupils over a long period.

Failure so early in acquiring such a highly valued skill as written language can thus have serious consequences. As mentioned, some children risk rapidly entering a vicious circle where defeats lead to new defeats. The chances of good learning decrease in step with the pupil's self-destructive attempts to avoid the written language. Some pupils become stubborn, noisy, aggressive, and lack concentration. Purely anti-social behaviour is not unusual. In some cases, there is an obvious risk of a criminal career.

Some recent Swedish investigations on prison clientele (Alm and Andersson, 1995; Levander and Lindgren, 1995) showed that a large proportion (about 65%) of the Swedish-speaking inmates had serious problems with reading and writing. In 60% of the prisoners, knowledge of spelling was below the average found in the 4th grade at school. In an American investigation (Newman et al., 1994), it was found that 75% of those in prison had serious reading and writing problems. In a Norwegian investigation of prison inmates, 20% reported that they had reading and writing problems (Tønnesen, 1995). In the last investigation, there were many who rejected the request to take part in the investigation. It is not unreasonable to suppose that many of these refused precisely because they had reading problems. The true figures of those with reading problems are therefore probably considerably higher.

It is often stated that a large proportion of prison inmates have dyslexia. It is argued that early defeats in such an important field as reading and writing as a result of dyslexia are so frustrating that they lead to aggression and behaviour problems in school. Failure can propel the pupil further in a vicious circle of new defeats and new types of behaviour problem, ending with anti-social behaviour, drug abuse, and criminality. A prison career has started.

One should be very careful with the interpretation here. It is probably true that many prison inmates have great difficulties with reading and writing, but it is more doubtful whether it is primarily a question of dyslexia. In a new investigation in Sweden (Samuelsson et al., forthcoming), it was assumed that dyslexia was a reasonable diagnosis if there were clear phonological problems. There were only 11 per cent of the inmates of a Swedish prison who had obvious phonological difficulties. However, the average level of the ability to read and write among the inmates was low, and could be compared with the mean level in pupils in the 6th grade. The difficulties with the written language were more likely to be the result of chaotic schooling and lack of stimulation and culture than the result of a dyslexic disposition. Reading is principally a cultural occupation, a skill that is developed, maintained, and refined in a cultural context. Prison inmates are often individuals who grow up under unfavourable conditions, and who are therefore deprived of the cultural capital necessary to make progress with the written language.

Regardless of the cause of the problems with reading and writing, they are a serious obstacle to those who try to adapt to a community and employment, which make great demands on the written language. A strategically important contribution to the rehabilitation process could be to give the inmates effective help aimed at improving their ability to read and write. Newman et al. (1994) refer to several studies that show that this type of training lessens the risk of recurrence.

In her thesis, Skaalvik (1994) has studied socioemotional problems and self-esteem in adults with reading and writing problems. She has let adults give an account of their time at school, and what effect this had on their later life. Skaalvik's work is important, especially because it concentrates on a qualitative understanding of the strategies that those with learning problems can develop in order to protect themselves from losing their self-esteem. Unfortunately, these strategies may make learning more difficult in the long run. There is a need of more thorough investigations of this kind.

Skaalvik's informants were taking part in adult education. They were particularly conscious of the pressure of work that occurred as a result of reading disabilities. Unpleasant experiences and bitter defeats from school life also rise to the surface under mental pressure. In this new attempt to become educated, it is important that these individuals spend much time on planning and choice of strategies that can facilitate learning. It should be noted that Skaalvik's informants were in the process of being educated. They probably represent a group which was not completely crushed by defeats at school. Even so, one suspects that many adults have had their belief in themselves as being capable of learning destroyed, and that their self-esteem is so damaged that they do not voluntarily begin a new education.

Assessment of possible emotional problems therefore becomes an important link in the diagnostic process.

By conversations with teacher and parents, and by systematic observations during the diagnostic process, an attempt is made to obtain a picture of emotional and motivational factors that may hinder learning to read. In some cases, it may also be relevant to consult psychological expertise and obtain a thorough analysis of the emotional and motivational aspects of the student.

Home environment

Some children come to school with several thousand hours fruitful contact with the written language behind them. The parents started early to read to their children, often as a bed-time ritual. The children have been given books as presents, played with plastic letters, received post-cards from their aunts and uncles, helped make shopping lists, learnt nursery rhymes, been encouraged to put their name on their drawings, in short taken many important steps in the development of their written language under informal conditions incorporated in play. They understand what writing is, they have an idea of the different functions of writing, they have become accustomed to the way information is packed into the written language, how words are arranged in sentences and paragraphs, and how sentences make a pattern that constructs a story. They have got to know a communication form that is not bound to *here and now*, but is independent of the situation. They have started to notice the form of words and understand that they can be divided into segments, and that different words can start with the same sound. They recognize a large number of the letters in the alphabet and can already read some simple words. The way into the written language will not be difficult for these children.

At the opposite extreme, we find children who are almost completely without familiarity with the written language from home. In these homes there are often no daily newspapers and there is a small number of books. (The IEA study showed that the number of books in a child's home was the single factor that had most influence on a child's reading skill.) The parents show absolutely no interest in reading. They never go to the library, never buy books, and only use written language when it is absolutely essential (Høien et al., 1994; Tønnessen, 1995).

Lack of access to the written language is not the only thing that characterizes these homes. It is also a question of 'atmosphere' in a more diffuse sense. The children are not expected to be good readers or bookworms. The parents do not function as models or identification figures as regards reading. Some parents may come from completely different cultures in other parts of the world where reading is not a highly valued activity. Meeting other people, conversations in cafés and public places may often be more important in this type of culture.

Children who grow up under these conditions often have a much more difficult passage into the written language. In these cases, the school has an enormous importance as a compensatory institution for the development of reading skill and pleasure in reading.

Insufficient instruction

In the great majority of pupils, learning to read is the result of systematic instruction. Negative conditions connected with instruction therefore represent serious obstacles. *Frequent changes of school* may have an especially negative effect on learning to read. The pupil may have been exposed to different methods without being able to develop a reliable method of decoding words. The result is often uncertainty and frequent guesses. *Frequent change of teacher* may have the same effect (Grogam, 1979).

Research affirms that quality class-room instruction in kindergarten and the primary grades is the best weapon against reading failure (National Research Council, 1998) Various *bad teaching habits* may increase the number of pupils with reading problems in a class. The following negative factors should be avoided. If the teacher:

1. fails to find out whether a pupil is ready to learn a new skill
2. uses too difficult teaching material
3. teaches too fast so that the pupil cannot follow
4. overlooks bad habits in the pupil's reading behaviour until they have become deeply rooted
5. overlooks the pupil and seldom asks him questions

6. gives little praise and encouragement
7. expresses displeasure and sarcasm if the pupil makes a wrong answer
8. permits, and even encourages, other pupils to disparage on fellow-pupils' achievements
9. expects a poor result from one pupil because his/her siblings were not clever
10. only uses one method in instructing beginners - not appropriate for all pupils

It is important to assess everything connected with the dyslexic's school and instruction conditions that may have made learning to read difficult. Conversations with the teachers, special teachers, school psychologist, parents, and the pupil him/herself will provide important information here.

Diagnosis of Adult Dyslexics

As with school pupils, the primary problem for adult dyslexics is localized at the word level. They have difficulty in rapidly and reliably recognising words, their spelling is poor, and there are not infrequently difficulties with syntax. The problem is particularly obvious when they try to read new words (Elbro et al., 1994; Pennington et al., 1990; Scarborough, 1984). This is also true when the IQ and socio-economic status are taken into account. The phonological awareness, and particularly the ability to deal with phonemes, is also poorly developed in adult dyslexics (Elbro et al., 1994; Felton et al., 1990; Kitz and Tarver, 1989). Elbro et al. (1994) have also shown that adult dyslexics may have indistinct or less precise articulation (diffuse knowledge of what words sound like when they are pronounced clearly). This manifests itself as less than clear speech in some dyslexics.

As we know, dyslexics have special problems in reading nonwords. Gross-Glenn et al. (1990) found that reading aloud of a text in which nonwords had been included could be used to diagnose dyslexia in adults. Normal readers stopped before nonwords and made certain that they managed to read them correctly, using the most usual rules of letter-to-sound conversion. The dyslexics used two different strategies. Some tried to read the text at the same speed as the normal readers, but mistakes were then frequent. Others reduced their speed of reading considerably to avoid making mistakes. Tests of the type used by Gross-Glenn should therefore be well-suited for diagnosing dyslexia in adults.

Mosberg and Johns (1994) investigated how much dyslexics understood of a text, both when they read the text themselves, and when an equally difficult text was read aloud to them. The object was to find out whether the problems of the dyslexics were specially connected with reading or whether there were more general problems in understanding language. It turned out that the dyslexics needed far more time than normal readers in connection with reading tasks. Comprehension was about the same in both groups. This supports other studies which also show that dyslexics above all need more time in order to reach the same level in reading comprehension as pupils without reading problems (see for example McLoughlin et al. 1994; Runyon, 1991).

Brief Summary

In order to diagnose dyslexia, one must include a thorough assessment of the word decoding strategies and of the separate processes behind the strategies. A thorough diagnosis of the dyslexic's spelling problems must also be carried out.

This assessment must be completed by an analysis of the pupil's linguistic functions (phonological and morphophonological awareness), an investigation of the reading comprehension, and an assessment of possible factors that may be obstructing the acquisition of reading and writing skills (poor intellectual ability, delayed language development, visual defects, impaired hearing, emotional/motivational problems, and unsatisfactory teaching). All diagnosis must take place with deep respect for the pupil as a fellow human being. Together, using different tests, we try to obtain greater insight into the strong and weak sides of the pupil, an insight on which educational remedial measures for the individual can be based.

CHAPTER 8

REMEDIATION

The poor reader often has to make a great effort to decode words. Reading becomes heavy going and exhausting, like bicycling against a head wind. Then it is important that the object of the journey is attractive. So many resources may be needed to decode words that there is no mental capacity left for comprehension processes. An important question in education therefore is to discover how to help the poor reader to acquire some automaticity in decoding. Compensatory techniques may also be a goal, for example books with cassette tapes, where the text has been recorded with clicks to indicate when you are supposed to turn the page. Some have found computer-based synthetic 'voices' that pronounce hard words a big help. Other measures to reduce the effort needed could include improving the visual, typographic, and linguistic design of the text. Informative illustrations may also be important.

The educational approach must take place on a broad front. It is not only a question of facilitating reading. It is also important to create a meaningful reading environment which the pupils experience as important and worthwhile. Another important factor is to choose texts which are felt to be personally significant, engaging, and relevant to the questions that interest young people, and which arouse emotions and invite identification.

Problems when Evaluating Remediation

In spite of the fact that educational measures are much used to help dyslexic pupils all over the world, only very rarely have these remedial measures been thoroughly and critically evaluated using scientifically acceptable methods. This is surprising, considering the prevalence of the dyslexia problem and the enormous resources used by special teachers. However, it is extremely difficult to assess the efficacy of an instruction programme. We will now discuss some of these difficulties.

The first problem is *regression toward the mean*. This is what we call the statistic effect that we often find when an individual has an extreme score in a test on one occasion: he tends to have a score nearer the mean next time the test is performed. This means that a dyslexic who has a low score in a reading test on one occasion will probably obtain a higher score next time, even though no supportive measures or treatment have been given. The regression effect may thus create the illusion that the pupil has made good progress in an effective educational programme when he hasn't. The statistical problem becomes even greater because many of the tests used in special education have very low reliability and diffuse objectives.

Another important problem when evaluating remedial measures is concerned with *the teacher's attitude*. The 'Hawthorne effect' is particularly problematic, i.e. teachers tend to greet with enthusiasm nearly any new method. Now, we know that enthusiastic teachers give their struggling pupils more attention and consideration when they employ a new method. So the improvement that we may see in the pupils is therefore not necessarily the result of the method alone, but surely reflects the teacher's new attitude to some degree. In connection with the large-major dyslexia project in Stavanger, Norway, we noticed a marked improvement in the reading scores of the dyslexics after the project had been going for a short time, even though the pupils had only been given a few tests. We think that parents and teachers imparted a positive and optimistic attitude to the pupils. In medicine we have the placebo effect: pills without any medically active ingredients bring about improvements of the condition. In order for such an effect to take place, the patient (and preferably also the doctor) must believe that it is an effective agent.

The teacher factor may also be difficult in other ways. If several teachers take part in trying out a new method, it may well be the case that some of them have developed or discovered the method and are enthusiastic about it, while others are skeptical, still others are indifferent or even negative to the project and participate only because the head teacher has said that everyone has to. Moreover, there is always the subtle interaction between teachers and pupils, and methods being tried out may therefore vary too much from class to class. An evaluation should thus include many classes so that these effects can be cancelled out.

It is surprising how rarely *control groups* are used in evaluation studies. Not having a control group makes it difficult at best to ascertain whether a method really has had an effect over and above what one would expect of the normal teaching. One of the reasons control groups are so seldom used is that a good control group should be selected at random. First you find a group of dyslexics, then you toss a coin or whatever to assign each dyslexic to either the control group or the study group. A *random selection* of this kind necessary for a causal analysis. But in special education investigations this raises the obvious ethical problem: If one believes that the programme being tested really is effective, it is morally difficult to deliberately exclude some pupils who might profit from it.

Other common weaknesses of investigations on the effects of treatment are that far too few pupils are followed for far too short a time with poorly specified programmes both as regards content and time spent. Another problem is that evaluation of progress is often made using tests that were standardized for normal readers. These tests may not be sensitive enough to pick up the small changes over short periods that we are interested in finding. This 'insensitive' instruments made it easy to underestimate the efficacy of many programmes.

Later in this chapter, when we discuss the different programmes or methods, we should remember that they have only very infrequently been subjected to strict scientific evaluation. This does not mean that they are of no value. Lengthy practical experience with the methods has shown that they seem to function. But it is desirable that someone had the time and resources to make a more thorough evaluation. The methods we present in this chapter are at any rate in good agreement with the theoretical foundation of dyslexia research as presented in this book.

General Principles of Educational Remediation in Dyslexics

Although research on special education encounters many methodological problems, it has been able to support some general principles of educational remediation in dyslexia. It is highly probable that dyslexics benefit from:

1. early identification and early help
2. basic phonological work
3. direct instruction
4. multisensory stimulation
5. mastery, overlearning, and automatization
6. good learning environment

Dyslexics have probably little benefit from:

1. waiting for the them to grow out of the problem
2. only providing extra attention and psychotherapy
3. punishment and threats
4. derogatory remarks such as *stupid, lazy, maladjusted*
5. visual and auditory perception training
6. several untraditional methods

We will now discuss some of the positive principles.

1. Early identification and early help

All teachers feel uneasy when they meet pupils in the lower primary school who are struggling with reading, and our worries increase when we see that the difference between poor and good readers steadily increases as the children move up in the school. The Matthew effect (the rich become richer and the poor become poorer) has been clearly documented (Stanovich, 1986).

Many of the pupils who stumble at the start may easily enter a vicious circle: Poor reading skills make all the subjects difficult. Some pupils thus easily lose faith in their own ability to learn, and some will unfortunately develop a negative attitude to school. Meeting poor readers in the lower primary school will always make experienced teachers reflect on the following questions: Is it possible to help these children, perhaps even before they know that they have a problem? Can we manage to start systematic measures at an early stage, before the pupil experiences failure and while the difference is still relatively small between those who succeed and those who have problems?

Recent research shows that we can help some of these pupils if we give them a real *push* at the start (Foorman et al., 1997). But this type of action necessitates willingness to think in new ways both as regards use of resources and planning instruction. Examples of special training programmes directed at first grade pupils at risk include 'Reading Recovery' (Clay, 1985), and 'First Steps' (Morris, 1995; Santa and Høien, 1999). These have given promising results and have led to pupils in the first grade making great progress, and the positive effect seems to persist as the pupils move up in the school (Wasik and Slavin, 1993). A strong and intensive effort in the first years of school may lead to a reduction in the pupil's need for resources for special education during the remainder of his/her school life. In the long term, this will save large sums of money for the school system. But the most important benefit of all is at the human level: In our opinion, if we succeed in lifting the individual pupils out of the vicious circle and over into more positive learning spirals, this in itself would be reason enough to offer these pupils qualified help and intensive and systematic training programmes

2. Basic phonological work

The basic problem in dyslexia is failure in the phonological system. We have also seen how phonological awareness is absolutely necessary in order to learn to read and write, and that dyslexics have particularly great problems with parsing words into phonemes and manipulating phonemes. It is thus natural to start by presenting remediation in this field.

Elkonin (1973) was one of the first to prepare an effective method for training phoneme parsing. Under a drawing of the word to be parsed, there are a series of empty boxes. The pupil is asked to articulate the word slowly. At the same time he draws a line in the box that corresponds to the sound he is articulating. The method has been evaluated in an investigation by Ball and Blachman (1988), where poor readers in the first grade were studied. In a subsequent follow-up, it was shown that the method was strikingly successful.

A Norwegian researcher who recognized the importance of phonological awareness earlier than most is Skjelfjord (1977). His training programme specially stresses the articulatory traits of the spoken word. Lie (1991) has followed this tradition and tried out training programmes in the first years of school, and these programmes have turned out to be successful (see Wise et al., 1990).

Well-controlled training studies have also been carried out in Sweden (Olofsson and Lundberg, 1985) and in Denmark (Lundberg et al., 1988). In these programmes, the children start with nursery rhymes. Rhyme exercises are thought to help children gain awareness of the form aspect of language. The children gradually started to analyze the sentences by clapping hands at each word, counting words, and indicating words with markers. The next step is concerned with morphemes in compound words and syllables. The word is parsed into these units and constructed again from the same units. Everything takes place as a game and in such a way that no-one feels he/she has failed the task. Phonemes are the critical step. Here one starts with an initial phoneme, first in short words with vowels, fricatives, and nasals. The plosive consonants (*b, d, g, p, t, k*), which are more strongly co-articulated and can't be sustained, come much later. When all the pupils understand how the initial phoneme is picked out, it is time to perform more thorough parsing. Progression is very slow, with frequent returns to an earlier step to make certain that all the pupils have understood. The programme has also been used individually in special education with very positive experiences. This programme has been translated and adapted to Americah preschools (Adams et al. (1998).

An interesting English investigation should be mentioned here: a training study reported by Bradley and Bryant (1985). The exercises included sorting pictures of words in categories. All the words resembled each other apart from one, for example *cat, mat, bat, pot, hat,* where *pot* does not fit. In some tests, the similarity was in the beginning of the word (alliteration), in others in the middle. One group worked with these exercises without letters, another group worked with plastic letters and were asked to show how they could write the words on the picture with these letters. A third group put the pictures into categories on the basis of semantic criteria, not phonological as in the first two groups, for example *horse, pig, car, dog,* where *car* does not fit. Finally, they had a fourth group who were not given any special offer. The results were very encouraging. The first two groups, who had phonological exercises, succeeded best in learning to read. Group 2, who had worked with letters, were best of all.

The investigations on phonological training referred to are very encouraging for work on the treatment of poor readers (Adams, 1990; Blachman, 1997; Borstrøm and Elbro, 1997; Lundberg, Olofsson and Wall, 1980; Torgesen et al., 1997; Wagner et al., 1994). They have the advantage of being well planned and well anchored in the theories on dyslexia. However, we still need more direct and long-term studies on the effect on the dyslexics (see also Niemi et al., 1999).

3. Direct instruction

Children generally seem to learn many things by being in a stimulating environment. It is as though knowledge and skills seep into them by osmosis. This osmosis does not seem to work in dyslexic pupils, at any rate as regards the written language. The pupil needs an adult who gives direct instruction, explains, points out, attracts attention, maintains interest and concentration.

Many investigations have shown that *time spent on learning* is of critical importance for progress. In ordinary classes, much time is spent on irrelevant matters, for example conflicts between pupils, practical tasks, waiting, day-dreaming, and so on. Dyslexics are particularly apt to use their time ineffectively, with long periods of unproductive waiting for help. The teacher is faced with a formidable problem of allotting time optimally between the pupils.

Dyslexic pupils thus need much direct guidance and much time in order to learn. This cannot always be achieved in an ordinary classroom environment. It is a good starting point for well-planned special education.

4. Multisensory stimulation

Multisensory stimulation includes teaching methods where several sensory channels are used during instruction. According to the definition, therefore, all instruction where speech is linked with visual symbols will be multisensory. However, the concept is normally assumed to cover methods based on an interaction between auditory, visual, kinaesthetic, and tactile modalities.

The kinaesthetic sense refers to movements of the body, while the tactile sense refers to the sense of feeling, for example by the fingertips. This is a sensory channel that is utilized to the maximum when blind people read Braille, but which is also stimulated by working with sandpaper letters, tracing in sand, and the like.

Tracing writing with the fingertips stimulates both the tactile and kinaesthetic senses. Tracing exercises are therefore an important component of the multisensory method.

Several multisensory techniques are based on Orton's theories (Orton, 1937). The idea behind the techniques was that one would compensate for weaknesses in the auditory or visual modality by instructing via other modalities. Instruction would be based on the pupil's strong points. Integration of information from different sensory modalities was assumed to build up new channels for acquiring reading and writing skills, and cooperation between the different sensory channels was important for the development of good reading and writing skills.

Several investigations on multisensory stimulation have been carried out. Hulme (1987) performed several interesting experiments to clarify the mechanisms behind multisensory learning. He considers that he has shown that tracing round forms increases the memory of these forms, and that the memory increase originates from activity in a separate motor memory system. Motor information also seems to be closely connected with visual memory. In the same way, the memory for articulatory movements is closely connected with auditory memory.

In word learning, the word is stored in the lexicon with a phonological, semantic, and orthographic identity in a reader with a developed reading skill. In a dyslexic, the phonological identities are diffuse, and the orthographic identities are often inaccurate or completely lacking. Another problem may be poorly developed association channels between the phonological and orthographic identities.

By means of multisensory stimulation, one can establish kinaesthetic, tactile, and articulatory identities for the word in the lexicon. Established identities can be bound to new-established identities in a network of association channels. The association channels are created by simultaneous stimulation of different sense modalities.

Learning letters is also a serious problem for many pupils when learning to read, particularly for many dyslexics. Both graphemes and phonemes are abstract units, the identity of which may be difficult to understand, and it may be difficult to associate the correct phoneme with the correct grapheme. The consequences of these difficulties may be confusion between letters. In order for knowledge of letters to function adequately when reading, the association channels have to function at an automatic level. Multisensory learning may strengthen the association through several association channels and contribute to automatization taking place more rapidly (Bradley, 1981; Simpson et al., 1992; Spear-Swerling and Sternberg, 1996).

In the same way, a network of identities and association channels can be created for other entities such as morphemes and syllables. Once a network of identities and association channels has been established in the lexicon, this system will continue to exist there. Activation of one of the identities will automatically lead to the other identities in the network being activated. The flow of information can thus follow several channels which simultaneously support each other. The multiplicity of identities will also function as sources of activation of the system.

A supplementary effect of multisensory stimulation will probably be that more attention is focused on the letter sequence in words, morphemes, and syllables, and on the characteristics of the letters.

There has been some criticism of multisensory stimulation, suggesting that there may be a danger of overstimulating the senses of the child. In practice, this has seldom been a problem. Even so, it has been shown that there is a small group of brain damaged children who develop problems when receiving information from several sensory channels simultaneously. In practice, one can take this into account by stimulating the sense modalities in pairs, thus building up the association network.

The use of other sense channels than the auditory and visual when teaching to read and write has long been known to have an effect both when teaching beginners and as a help for pupils with reading and writing problems. Multisensory stimulation has therefore formed the basis of many methods.

5. Mastery, overlearning and automatization

In an ordinary classroom, teaching progresses in relation to the achievement level of the average pupil. The teacher moves on when he thinks that most of the pupils have reached a reasonable level of mastery. Most of the pupils have by then also received a certain amount of overlearning, which means that they remember as learning proceeds. This does not apply to dyslexics in subjects that are based on written language. They fail here, partly because they never get the chance of reaching a mastery level. They then forget the acquired skills more easily than their fellow pupils and proceed into new phases with a poor foundation.

Earlier in this book we have mentioned the importance of decoding becoming automatic. This means that it is encapsulated into a well-functioning module which does not need attention and does not drain resources from the important job of interpretation. Dyslexics need a particularly long time before word decoding has become automatic. They need much more practice than normal readers. As mentioned previously, many dyslexics soon enter a vicious circle where they have learnt to avoid reading, which becomes another obstacle to acquiring good skills. The great educational challenge is now to *break the vicious circle*. There are no simple solutions here. Patience, sensitivity, and understanding are needed; it is important to demonstrate that mastery can give pleasure and satisfaction; it is important to awaken a love of reading; it is important to make the pupil believe in him/herself (Dougherty and Johnston, 1996).

It is not easy to achieve all this in a normal classroom. Nor is it easy with one or two hours special education a week, specially when these hours are taken from the regular language instruction, or when the dyslexic is taken out of lessons where he/she experiences some success, for example domestic science, arts and crafts, etc. Illnesses, leisure time, sport, and other activities at school also tend to reduce the time allotted for special education substantially. In Denmark, new forms of organization for teaching dyslexics have been tried. *Reading courses*, a concentrated, intensive instruction period where 12-15 hours a week are set aside for reading and writing instruction, have given good results. In principle, many of the guidelines mentioned above can be followed here. Experience of this organization model has been very positive. When considering remediation, one needs to be aware of the various methods of organizing instruction.

Repeated reading

One method that is used to promote automatic decoding skill is *repeated reading*, which means that the pupil reads the same text several times. The effect of repeated reading is generally good (Dowhower, 1994), but the benefit naturally varies from one pupil to another. Some pupils think that repeated reading is boring and not very motivating. They recognise the text, and the reading itself does not present them with any new content. However, the method may have a positive effect on reading development in other pupils. It will therefore be up to the individual teacher to assess to what extent the method is suitable for each pupil. In order to make repeated reading more motivating, it is important to include an element of competition in the reading. The object is to see whether repeated reading results in progress as regards fewer reading errors (checked by the teacher) and increased speed of reading (checked by the pupil with a stop watch). The pupil is given a form where he/she fills in the number of words read correctly and the time taken to read the text. The results can then be transferred to a diagram that shows progress. Many pupils are familiar with diagrams of this kind when training for sport, and they therefore enjoy using a similar procedure with reading. If this method is to function, it is important that the teacher chooses the length, content, and degree of difficulty with care. Poor readers give up easily if the material is too difficult. Then it is better to start with reading material that is too easy (Layton and Koenig, 1998).

Alternating reading

Another method that seems to work very well in poor readers is *alternating reading*, which means that both teacher and pupil are involved during reading. The starting point is that both teacher and pupil have the same text, and that the text is chosen carefully to suit the individual pupil. It is important that the teacher starts by reading one or two pages of the book, adjusting the reading speed to the pupil's reading skill, so that the pupil can follow the text during the reading process.

Once the teacher has read 1-2 pages, he suggests that the pupil should read a little, perhaps two or three lines. Now the teacher has the *pupil role*, i.e. he or she must follow the text as the pupil reads. This alternating reading continues, but the teacher gradually reduces his own reading while the pupil reads more. An agreement can also be made whereby the teacher and pupil will read a given number of lines each.

Then comes the stage that the pupil likes best, and which provides best possibilities for games and variation. The teacher and pupil agree that the teacher will read as many lines as he likes, and he often stops in the middle of a sentence. The pupil then continues to read as long as he likes. When the pupil stops, it is the teacher's turn. This continues until the text has been read through. It is important that the pupil is allowed to choose how much he/she wants to read, as adjustments can then be made depending on how the pupil feels that day and motivation. If the pupil only chooses to read short pieces of text, the teacher must find out why this is so. Sometimes the pupil may be trying to get out of reading. Then the teacher himself can read short sections, so that the pupil has to read again soon. But if the pupil is trying as hard as he can, but is tired and not motivated, he is rewarded by the teacher reading more, and the pupil is allowed to read less. Experience has shown that it is rare for the pupil not to follow the text if it has attracted his interest, and if the degree of difficulty is appropriate to the pupil's reading skill.

In order for alternating reading to succeed, it is essential to choose the right texts, where the choice depends on the interests and reading level of the pupil.

Chorus reading and pair reading

Chorus reading is another variant used in reading training which many poor readers find safe and therefore acceptable. Chorus reading implies that a whole group of pupils read the text together. In this way, the poor reader does not stand out, but gains a feedback from the others when he meets a word that he/she does not recognise (Topping and Parkinson, 1996).

Pair reading may be appropriate in group teaching of poor readers. There are then two pupils who read alternately. The one who is not reading is the *teacher* who follows the text and checks to see whether the reader makes any mistakes. A stop watch to record speed of reading can also be used here.

The text that has been read can be used as a basis for talking about the text, explaining words and concepts that are not known, reflecting on the text, and so on.

6. Good learning environment

A good learning environment is of obvious importance (Scanlon and Vellutino, 1997; Vellutino et al., 1997). In order to illustrate the importance of a good learning environment on children learning to read, we will present the results obtained by two large research studies carried out by The National Reading Research Center in USA. These studies focused on what characterizes a good environment for learning to read:

One of the studies focused on conditions in a kindergarten, and 1st and 2nd grade (ordinary classes) (Pressley et al., 1996), and another study included special education (Rankin and Pressley, forthcoming).

In each investigation, the teachers were asked to write down the ten factors that they considered were most important in order to create a good environment for learning to read. Their answers formed the basis of a survey investigation in which teachers were asked to state an opinion on a number of statements. A total of 89 teachers and 34 special teachers took part in the investigation. They were all experienced reading teachers of long standing who were known for their good results in teaching to read. The eight most important characteristics of a good environment for learning to read are given below:

1. Abundant reading material in the classroom (many books of varying degree of difficulty)
2. Emphasis on both skill training (e.g. phonological awareness, phonological synthesis, etc.) and frequent reading of children's books
3. Varied forms of reading (repeated reading, chorus reading, reading to oneself)
4. Varied reading material (stories, technical texts, poems, easily read books)
5. Explicit instruction in the writing process (process oriented writing)
6. Same elements in the instruction for both poor readers and those who read well. However, poor readers need more:
   explicit training in phonological skills (including phonological awareness),
   explicit training in word decoding,
   more teacher-directed instruction
7. Make reading pleasant (motivated reading)
   reduce the risk of failure
   much positive feedback
   make the pupils believe that they will succeed in learning to read
8. Follow up the pupils' progress in reading and writing
   assessments use of portfolios (selection of work done by pupils, which is gone through with the teacher during separate sessions) meetings with parents

In order to succeed in putting these items into practice, it is essential that the school's teachers have sufficient knowledge of reading and writing disabilities. That is why it is so important that both instruction and practice in this field should be included in the basic training of those learning to be teachers. This has also been strongly emphasized in the report by The Orton Dyslexia Society (1997): 'Informed instruction for reading success: Foundations for teacher preparation.' Here, it is stressed how important it is that the basic training of pre-school and primary school teachers should include extensive information on reading, reading development and problems, and practical training in how to help pupils with reading and writing disabilities. Only then do we obtain 'informed instruction', which is essential for 'reading success'.

The authorities should enable teachers who have not received the necessary special education in their basic training to update their knowledge by offering refresher courses.

However, knowledge alone is not enough to ensure a really good learning environment. Many other factors are also necessary. We particularly stress how important it is that the pupils should have their basic needs for security and affection satisfied, and that the instruction is organized so that they experience success: 'Nothing succeeds like success'.

All effective methods are permeated by warm personal relations between pupil and teacher. When the pupil experiences the teacher as someone who *cares*, who shows confidence and warmth, there is a dramatic increase in the chances of development and learning. There is much to indicate that the successful methods give results because they give room for one-to-one tuition of the pupil by the teacher. One-to-one tuition increases the chances of time on task, intensity, perseverance, and willingness to learn. But above all, it gives room for confidence, engagement, and reciprocity (for survey see Baker et al., 1996; Guthrie and Wigfield, 1997; Hall and Moats, 1999; Tuley, 1998).

Remediation to Promote Decoding Skill

Learning reliable knowledge of letters

Most pupils do not find it particularly difficult to learn letters. By reading frequently, their knowledge of letters becomes established in a natural manner. However, this is not so easy for dyslexics. Learning letters is therefore an important part of the instruction of poor readers. After the pupil has learnt the ordinary letter-sound combinations, teaching unfortunately often fails to continue with the sounds (phonemes) that really are complicated for dyslexic pupils. We have in mind the phonemes that do not correspond with a single letter, but where several letters have to be used to portray the sound (e.g. *sh, sch, ch, ng,* etc.). But it is precisely these grapheme-phoneme correspondences that instruction should emphasize most.

The pupil also has to learn to recognize how consonant clusters are articulated (e.g. *tr, cr, pr,* etc.), and much attention should be paid to recognizing frequently occurring letter sequences either as prefixes, suffixes, or sequences in the middle of a word. We call this the 'analogy strategy': teaching the pupil that some patterns are found in a great many words, and that it is useful to recognize these letter patterns so that they do not have to sound out a word when only one letter differs from a previously learnt word. We can also speak of using the metacognitive strategy to teach the pupil an effective word decoding strategy. Although most pupils acquire this knowledge more or less unconsciously through repeated encounters with words, some pupils need explicit introduction into how it can be done.

Learning reliable associations between orthographic and phonological units

Starting with single letters when reading unknown words is a laborious decoding strategy. Good reading skills are characterized by the readers immediately being able to recognize larger elements of the word, for example syllables, morphemes, or the word as a whole. Most readers acquire this orthographic knowledge almost regardless of reading method. Many dyslexics seem to have got stuck in a laborious sounding out strategy, and this strategy prevents them from acquiring orthographic knowledge at a higher level (Peterson and Haines, 1992).

How can one best help such pupils? It seems clear that in pupils with great phonological difficulties, it is very important to learn how letter patterns and words can be recognized without resorting to sounding out first. This means that the teacher must put a lot of work into getting the pupil to recognize sequences of letters, whether they are syllables, morphemes, or whole words. One approach which functions well with many poor readers is to work with *word families* (see Santa and Høien, 1999). The words *house, mouse,* and *louse* all belong to the same family because they have something in common, i.e. the letter sequence *-ouse*. The main point is that the pupil will discover that there is a system in word recognition. Most of the new words that the pupil meets resemble other words that he/she already knows. What the pupil has to learn is that he/she must consciously start using this knowledge. Spelling can be confusing, but there is some method to its madness. Much has been written on the significance of metacognition in connection with reading comprehension, and it is an important subject. But it is also important to focus on how important it is for poor readers to learn effective metacognitive strategies in connection with the word decoding process, for example conscious use of the analogy strategy (Goswami and Mead, 1992; Seymour and Evans, 1994).

Learning reliable and automatic word decoding

In order to have a good reading skill, it is essential that the reader recognizes most words immediately, i.e. he or she has acquired a large number of ready-for-use orthographic identities. Poor readers often have a very limited repertoire of ready-for-use identities, hence their laborious decoding. Fast and reliable word decoding skill comes as a result of reading a lot. It is important that the teacher finds reading matter that matches the reading skill of the pupil, and that he/she awakens a love of reading. It is also important to inform the parents of the significance of children's reading outside school hours or in connection with homework.

It is important that acquiring ready-for-use word identities can take place in an atmosphere that is as similar as possible to a game, and that unnecessary mechanical repetition is avoided. One exercise that has been shown to function very well for poor readers is a word-card game. Several sets of words are prepared that the pupils will learn to recognize on sight, for example 8 pairs of words. The words are written in block letters on pieces of cardboard (4 x 4 cm), and to start with, the pupils learn to recognize these words. The aim is that the pupil should learn to recognize the words as pictures, but this is based on precise instruction by the teacher, who shows how the letter sequences in the word make it possible to recognize it. A conscious effort is made to avoid allowing the pupil to try to recognize the word on the basis of more or less random visual characteristics (see logographic reading in Chapter 2). It is therefore most advantageous that the words selected for training do not differ from each other too much orthographically.

The word-cards are then divided into two heaps, and the teacher and pupil present the words to each other one at a time. When the teacher reads the pupil's card, it is the pupil who assesses whether the answer is correct or not. When the teacher holds out a card it is the pupil's turn, and the teacher decides whether the answer is correct. In order to create some excitement, the teacher can throw in some deliberate misreadings - to ensure that the pupil is paying attention.

After the pupil has worked with single words for a period, the teacher can suggest that they play Concentration. The cards are shuffled and laid out face down on the table in a square pattern. The pupils starts by drawing two cards. He then has to decide whether they match. If they are, the pupil gains one point and can draw two more cards. If the words are not a pair they are put back in the same place. Now it is the teacher's turn. The game continues until all the pairs of words have been found. The player with most pairs has won.

If the pupil is weak, the teacher should let the pupil win at first. As the pupil's skill increases, the teacher may well find it difficult to beat the pupil - young children are often pretty good at remembering locations. The number of pairs of words is gradually increased, and the teacher can keep word-card pairs in plastic bags of varying degrees of difficulty.

A combination of sound method and whole word method

The two best known reading methods in most countries are the *sound method* ('phonics') and the *whole word method* (whole language*)*. The sound method is based on learning grapheme-phoneme associations, and by combining the sounds the pupil discovers which word has been written. The whole word method is based on the pupil learning several words as complete visual identities. In basal readers it is rare that only one method is used, though the relative emphasis on method may vary from one textbook to another.

Most pupils learn to read no matter which method is used. Instruction is probably best if elements from both methods are used. If these two main methods are combined in a sensible way and notice is taken of the individual pupil's needs and abilities, we believe that this provides the optimum chance of more pupils succeeding in learning to read. It is always possible that a one-sided and perhaps misconceived use of a given instruction method - no matter how good it is - may cause reading problems. The International Reading Association (IRA) therefore recommends a balanced approach in reading instruction (Pressley et al., 1996, Rankin and Pressley, forthcoming). Moreover, we refer to what has previously been written in the section 'Good learning environment' in this chapter.

Technical Aids that can be Used to Promote Reading Skill

Books with cassettes

Books with cassettes consist of a printed text with an accompanying tape recording. The text on the tape is identical to the printed text. The tape and book are used together, so that the pupil listens to the recorded text and follows the words on the page *at the same time*. This is primarily an educational tool for enhancing reading skill. The text must be simple, and the reading must be slow and clear enough so that the pupil can read the text and understand the content. In order to adjust the reading to pupils at different skill levels, it is often necessary to read the same text at different speeds.

The slow readers, and those who lack concentration, often associate reading with a very unpleasant situation. They seldom get far enough into a book to become engaged by it. When they neither can nor want to read, they do not obtain the practice necessary for progression. Books with cassettes have given good results in this relatively large group. There are many instances where this approach helped to break the vicious circle and open the way for progress. If the reading difficulties are due to lack of reading or language training, books with cassettes may well help.

Experience has shown that books with cassettes do not only improve reading skill in these groups, but also improves their ability to listen and concentrate. At the same time, the children get beneficial training in auditory, visual, and motor functions. The pupil hears (auditory), sees (visual) and pronounces (motor) the words in the text and can safeguard the connections between the different modalities by following the text with a finger (Glezheiser and Clark, 1991).

Some have feared that cassettes and books would create dependence, so that children learn to listen *instead* of reading. Experience has shown that this does not happen. When the pupil discovers that his eyes can run faster through the text than the voice on the tape, he generally prefers to read himself.

Computer-based training

Several computer programmes have been developed to help reading and writing disabilities. Selection of type of programme naturally depends on which reading and writing disability is present. There are many programmes adapted to individual needs. It is possible to adjust the procedure as the pupil progresses and new needs arise. One big advantage of many of these programmes is that the pupil can always get feedback about his/her results. The unlimited possibilities for repetition are also important.

A programme that stresses metacognitive content has been used with success in Umeå in Sweden. This programme is based on an American programme from Colorado (Olson and Wise, 1992), and it works like this (see also Lundberg and Olofsson, 1993; Poskiparta, Vauras and Niemi, 1998).

The reader chooses a text from a menu. The text appears on the computer screen. When the reader encounters a word that is difficult to identify, he can ask for help by marking the word. The word is then highlighted, and an artificial voice gives the pronunciation. Either the whole word is pronounced, or the student can ask for parts of the word, for example syllable by syllable or phoneme by phoneme. The advantage of synthetic speech is that just about all the words in the texts that are fed into the machine can be pronounced without having to wait. The reader can thus get immediate and effective help while reading, even though the voice does sound a bit artificial.

A computer can register and store the words that the pupil has marked, and also calculate out how long it took to read the page of text, how many words were marked on each page, and which words. An important advantage of this method is that it gives the pupil control over his own reading. There are no words that cannot be identified easily and quickly. In ordinary texts, the dyslexic pupil is at great risk of meeting words that he does not completely succeed in reading.

Secondly, a computer can give the dyslexic pupil an opportunity of reading texts that are above the level that he can really master, but with a content that is more suitable for his level. Practically all texts can be scanned into the computer, complete with any accompanying pictures and diagrams. This allows the programme to be used outside of school as well (Wise et al., 1997).

Reading with help from a computer allows the pupil has to supervise his own reading continuously. (This is the metacognitive component.) The programme 'forces' the pupil to continuously assess whether or not to ask for help from the artifical voice. Most dyslexics have not really developed the knack for knowing when they need help and when they don't. Instead, they've often got into the habit of simply skipping over the difficult words and hoping that things will sort themselves out. Being able to ask for help from a computer - without embarrassment or fear of boring the 'teacher', allows them to learn *when* they need help. This in turn increases their metacognitive ability. These types of computer programmes can help break down a passive and despairing attitude and help the pupil realise that he can control his own reading progress.

Computer training also allows students to read connected, self-selected, and meaningful texts. Attention gets focused on content and meaning, which after all is the 'real world' point of reading. Building decoding skills is merely a by-product, as indeed it is merely a by-product of 'normal' students' reading.

Methods and Programmes which can Prevent and Remedy Decoding Difficulties

We will take a closer look at five different reading methods/programmes which have been shown to give good results in instructing poor readers: Fernald's VAKT method, The Orton/Gillingham/Stillman method, The Lindamood Auditory Discrimination in Depth programme, Reading Recovery, and Early Steps. We will give most space to the Early Steps programme, which has been shown to be very effective in preventing and remedying serious reading disabilities.

Fernald's VAKT method

Grace Fernald's ideas were conceived in the first half of this century. She had no explicit theory behind her work, but it seems that she considered memory for movements as being very important. Fernald's pupils were of different ages, but they all had great reading and writing problems. Clinical experience showed that her method gave positive results (Fernald, 1943).

VAKT stands for the interaction between Visual, Auditive, Kinaesthetic, and Tactile stimulation. Emphasis on recognition of words, for example by tracing exercises, is an important component of Fernald's method. The pupil acquires knowledge of the shape of the letter by feeling letter shapes or tracing letters cut out of sandpaper. Another characteristic of the method is emphasis on natural motivation. Research shows that Fernald's method is effective in the instruction of dyslexic pupils (Spear-Swerling and Sternberg, 1996).

The Orton/Gillingham/Stillman method

Gillingham and Stillman were amongst the earliest pioneers in multisensory techniques (1969, 1st edition from the 1930s). In The Orton/Gillingham/Stillman method, the pupil works with letters, sequences of letters, analysis of sequences of letters, analysis of regular words, and finally analysis of longer and more complicated words. The method is based on interaction between visual, auditive, kinaesthetic, and tactile learning. When learning to be aware of phonemes, the pupil learns how the sound is formed in the mouth, and supporters of the programme maintain that this reinforces learning of the letters. In the next step, the name of the letter is included to attract attention to the sequence of letters in words. Research shows that this method is useful for many dyslexic pupils (Lindamood, Bell and Lindamood, 1997; Schupack and Wilson, 1997).

The Lindamood Auditory Discrimination in Depth programme

This method is based on the Orton/Gillingham/Stillman method, but puts even more emphasis on systematic practising of phonemic awareness, training in phoneme analysis, and use of articulatory factors in connection with phoneme learning and in discrimination of sound-related phonemes (Lindamood and Lindamood, 1975).

Research shows that this method functions well in pupils with great reading disabilities (see Byrne and Fielding-Barnsley, 1995; Torgesen, Wagner and Rashotte, 1997).

The Reading Recovery programme

The Reading Recovery programme aims at helping pupils who, after 12 months of traditional instruction, still have great reading difficulties (Clay, 1985). The programme regards reading as a psycholinguistic process where the reader constructs meaning on the basis of the text. The programme contains the following subcomponents: Perceptual analysis, knowledge of the conventions of the written language ('print awareness'), decoding, verbal language training, emphasis on previous knowledge, reading strategies, and metacognition (Wasik and Slavin, 1993). The instruction is given daily, each training session lasts 30 minutes, and always in the form of one-to-one tuition. The teachers have all had special instruction in the use of the Reading Recovery method. The fundamental principle behind the method is that reading is a strategic process, that reading and writing are activities which are strongly connected, and that the pupils should be engaged in much reading of relevant texts (Wasik and Slavin, 1993). A typical training session could consist of the following activities:

1.   reading from two or more books which the child has already read at least once before
2.   independent reading from the book that was introduced the day before
3.   learning letters
4.   writing a story that the child has composed alone. Here, emphasis is put on analysis of phonemes in the word (using Elkonin's 'box' method, 1973)
5.   cutting up a text into single words, which are then put together to form a text again
6.   introducing a new book
7.   reading from the new book

Reading Recovery is much used in New Zealand, USA, and Canada. More information on the Reading Recovery programme can be found in Center et al. (1995). Several evaluations of the effect of Reading Recovery have been carried out (Hiebert, 1994; Spiegel, 1995; Pinnell et al., 1994). One of the criticisms of the programme has been that it puts too little emphasis on systematic introduction of phonological skills, which have been demonstrated by research to be important in promoting learning to read (Chapman and Tunmer, 1993). Iversen and Tunmer (1993) compared the effect of two somewhat different versions of Reading Recovery. In one version they put more emphasis on systematically presented phonological skills. The results showed that this type of modification gave significantly better results than the traditional Reading Recovery programme.

The Early Steps programme

Santa (1995) gives a detailed description of the training programme 'Early Steps'. Research shows that the programme has a good effect (Santa and Høien, 1999).

The pupils who are selected for inclusion in testing 'Early Steps' are selected after systematic assessment (Morris and Perney, 1994; Morris, 1992). The training programme gives each pupil about 30 minutes one-on-one instruction every day, either by the class teacher or by a special teacher. The pupils are taken out of the class for their lessons. Most pupils need between 45 and 60 hours before they can read well enough to 'graduate' the programme. Each training session contains four basic components:

1.   repeated reading from known books
2.   writing sentences
3.   sorting letters or words
4.   presentation of a new book

1. Repeated reading from known books

Structured reading periods with an experienced teacher can help the students understand how they can predict happenings/content of a text on the basis of title and pictures. The pupils can learn to think about what they should pay attention to while reading, and the reading helps them to develop a larger and more active vocabulary. These factors represent experience and knowledge which we know can contribute to increasing reading comprehension (Stanovich, 1996).

2. Writing sentences

The teacher starts by asking the pupil to write a sentence based on own experiences and interests. The sentence is then used in different forms of phonological analysis training. This activity is well known from traditional special education. Once the pupil has decided what he/she is going to write, the teacher and pupil find out together how many and which words the sentence consists of. The pupil is then encouraged to write down the sentence word for word. Phonological analysis skills at the phoneme level are necessary in order to identify the sounds in the words. Knowledge of letters must be activated when these sounds are linked to the corresponding graphemes. Use of Elkonian letter 'boxes' when writing difficult words may help the pupil to become aware of how many sounds there are in the word.

3. Sorting letters or words

Part of the problem for pupils who struggle with reading is that they cannot manage to transfer knowledge from one word to another. When they read they attack each new word as though they had never seen anything like it before. They need to learn to make their reading more efficient, by utilizing the information contained in the graphic pattern of the words: When they've learnt to read *cat*, they should not struggle with *hat* and *rat*.

We need to increase their awareness of the patterns of words, so that they will be able to transfer their hard-won knowledge from one word to other words that share the same pattern. 'Early Steps' uses word-sorting tasks to develop this awareness. In this training sequence, the pupil is asked to sort word cards into 'families' of different types: words that start with the same sound, words that end with the same sound, words that have the same vowel-sound in the middle, and words that start or end with the same letter-sequence, and the like. It is important to start the sortings at a level that the pupil masters. Usually this will be sorting the word cards into families by their initial sounds. The teacher naturally has to help out so that the pictures are put into the correct piles, but it is just as important that the pupil is helped to understand *why* the placing is correct.

Gradually, as the teacher sees that the pupil easily manages to sort word cards by the first sound, it is important that she presses the pupil on to the next level: sorting by the last sound, then middle vowel, and finally sorting by more complicated criteria, such as initial or final letter-sequence.

Word sorting is an activity that has been shown to be very effective, specially for pupils with major phonological problems. One explanation of why sorting seems to help is that it gets the pupil to direct his attention to written and spoken identities simultaneously. In this way, the orthographic/visual and phonological/auditory patterns mutually reinforce each other (Santa and Høien, 1999).

4. Presentation of a new book

Each training session finishes with the introduction of a new book, hopefully one that is at just the right level of difficulty for the student. Together, the teacher and pupil go through the book, look at the pictures, identify difficult words, and read the text together by alternate reading or echo reading. Conversations between the teacher and pupil on the new books also provide a good way of demonstrating how the pupil can learn to ask good metacognitive questions (Pramling, 1988). We can thus show the pupil how he/she can benefit from his/her own experience and background knowledge during the reading process.

'Early Steps' is resource-demanding in many respects. Most schools will find it difficult (or even impossible) to carry out the programme for 'normal poor readers' in the lowest grades. Since we know that elements of the programme have such a positive effect on learning to read, we must see whether they can be adapted and used in ordinary teaching.

In many other countries, 6 and 7 year-olds are seldom taken out of class for intensive special instruction. This type of remedial work is commonly reserved for very special cases, and is perhaps most often used with pupils who have other educational goals than 'normal' pupils.

We also have certain reservations against introducing systematic screening of 6 year-olds if the object is to pick out a group of pupils who will receive intensive special education from the first months of the first grade. It would be better to use the ideas in 'Early Steps' in normal teaching. Ideally, the principles and assumptions found in 'Early Steps' should be part of the process of learning to read from the start.

On the basis of experience in the trial of 'Early Steps' (and other similar training programmes), Engen (1996) recommends that a training programme for poor readers in the second grade should be based on the following principles:

1. The training programme is offered and developed for individual pupils on the basis of thorough and systematic individual assessment

2. It is essential that the learning environment is safe and supportive. The pupil must feel that he/she succeeds in the different parts of the training programme

3. The teacher must be well qualified and know both the pupil and about reading and writing problems

4. The programme for each pupil should be planned so that there is slow but clear progression. The pupil must be given time and a reassuring atmosphere so that he/she can consolidate his/her knowledge and has a chance of registering progress

5. The best results are obtained when the pupil understands that there is a connection between the teaching material (choice of books

etc.) in the training programme and in the regular classroom instruction
6.   Reading books must be an important part of the programme. Some of the books should be new, others the pupil should have already read at least once before
7.   The pupil's skill in reading words should be increased and become automatic

At first glance, a training programme like 'Early Steps' may seem rather exclusive: thorough assessment, one-to-one tuition by well qualified teachers for 25-30 minutes every day for almost a whole school year. It is easy to imagine that ideas like this may be met with arguments such as: 'We cannot afford this. This would be impossible to carry out - at any rate in our school'. To these reactions we would reply by asking: 'Can we afford not to try?' The vicious circle poor readers wind up in also costs a lot, both in money and in the form of non-quantifiable personal problems.

Measures to Promote Reading Comprehension

Dyslexic pupils are generally given far too little practice in reading for comprehension. Their instruction has necessarily focused on decoding. The danger in this is that many dyslexics come to believe that reading is primarily a question of recognizing words correctly, and not an activity that aims at finding the meaning of a text. However, it is not easy to teach reading comprehension. In an investigation on reading instruction in some grades in USA, Durkin (1978-79) found that of 17,997 minutes of direct reading instruction, less than 50 minutes were spent on instruction in reading comprehension.

There are now several investigations that directly demonstrate the effect of metacognitive training programmes in strategies to promote reading comprehension among dyslexics. We will now look at the significance of some of these strategies.

Learning new words

Many poor readers have a poorly developed vocabulary because they read little and lack good strategies to develop their vocabulary. They are also trapped in a vicious circle that can be very difficult to break out of. Children can learn the meaning of many new words if the words are in a meaningful context or if they are explained. The new words become part of the children's property by being linked to experiences that the children themselves have had. It is important that instruction gives the children an open, flexible, and multi-dimensional attitude to language, so that they are able to realize that a word can have different meanings according to which context it appears in. Instruction must also awaken the pupils' interest in the new words they meet in the text. It has been estimated that on average, pupils learn 3,000 new words a year. Obviously, all these words cannot be learnt through the teacher's instruction. Most of them the pupil has learnt on her own. It is therefore important to ask what we can do to teach the children a strategy so that they are able to develop their vocabulary to a maximum extent, via their encounters with the writing.

A traditional approach when teaching new words has been that the teacher explains the new words *before* the pupil starts to read the text. However, one should be careful not to overwork this approach. The problem is, that when words are taken out of their context and 'defined', the whole exercise becomes very abstract and academic. Do students really remember these definitions? And if they do, have we denied them the chance to figure out the meaning of an unfamiliar word from the context? We want them to have capacious vocabularies, but perhaps even more than that we want them to be able to *acquire* rich vocabularies on their own. If the student is going to learn 3,000 words this year, and the teacher only has time to present a mere handful per week, obviously we need to impart to children the skills necessary to figure things out on their own.

Research has shown that the vocabulary of dyslexic pupils increases much faster if the traditional dictionary-type definition of the word is replaced by thorough explanation of the meaning of the word (Weisberg, 1988). This approach is also best for pupils with normal reading skills (Pressley et al., 1989).

Background knowledge

The background knowledge that the reader has when he meets a text has a decisive effect on whether he will understand the content of the words and the meaning of the text as a whole. 'World knowledge' is important in order to obtain 'word knowledge'. Letters and words do not in themselves have content. It is not until the words meet a reader who seeks meaning that they obtain their content. Children cannot read with comprehension unless they can relate the new information in the text to the background knowledge that they already possess.

Preparing a text by long *conversations* where the teacher draws connections with the child's experiences, seems like a waste of time. But time is not really wasted if ideas and concepts that help the child to interpret the text are developed and made relevant. It is like giving the child a 'map'. Dyslexic pupils do not always realize that there is any connection between what they read and what they already know. But if they are given background information on the main character or the most important ideas in a text before they start to read, there is less risk that they get onto the wrong track or become confused by the text. Instead, the chances increase that they will understand the story completely. When they take part in thought-provoking discussions before the story starts, it is also easier for them to understand that the object of reading is to gain knowledge, experience and insight, and not merely to decipher the words on the page. Research has shown that even pre-school children can be trained to make metacognitive reflections such as 'Why am I doing this?', 'Why do you think we are doing this?', and so on (Pramling, 1988).

The grammar and metacognition of the story

In a narrative text, it is possible to draw a 'map' of the events, depicting the main characters and events in a causal chain. This knowledge of the structure of the story, the *story grammar*, makes it easier for the reader to understand the text. Knowledge of how the story is constructed will also help the pupil to compose his/her own stories. It is important to give dyslexics metacognitive insight into the structure of different texts. This is difficult for dyslexics, but research has shown that systematic instruction in story grammar increases reading comprehension (Cain, 1996; Reiff et al., 1994).

Use of visual representations of the main ideas in a story, asking questions related to the text, and making summaries are all examples of metacognitive comprehension strategies (see Aaron, forthcoming). In many cases, several of these strategies are combined in individual comprehension programmes, and we will now give an account of three of the best known programmes.

Programmes for Promoting Reading Comprehension

We will give a brief account of three programmes: 'Explicit instruction', 'Reciprocal instruction' and the 'CRISS programme'.

Explicit instruction

This programme is described by Pearson and Leys (1985). The teacher bases the teaching on a specific strategy, for example drawing conclusions (inferences), and chooses reading material to teach this strategy. He then shows four processes that will be used during reading: (1) asking a question (in this case a inference-type question); (2) answering the question, which means that one has to read a sentence or a whole text; (3) finding support in the text for the answer; (4) explaining one's thoughts and reasoning. When the teacher has demonstrated these four processes thoroughly, the pupil attempts to solve the problems alone by answering the last two items (finding support in the text for the answer and explaining his/her own thoughts). The next step can be that the teacher asks the inference question and points out where in the text the relevant information can be found. The pupil has to provide the answer. The next step is that the teacher only asks the question, and the pupil takes care of the other items from (2) to (4). Finally, the pupil takes over responsibility for the whole sequence.

Later modifications of this method also include a sequence where the pupil is asked to discuss experiences that resemble events in the text. The pupil is also encouraged to say what he thinks will happen next in the story. An investigation carried out by Hansen and Pearson (1983) showed that poor readers in the 4th grade benefited far more from this than normal readers, who found the exercises boring.

Reciprocal instruction

Reciprocal instruction is a particularly interesting method for training strategies with dyslexic pupils (Palinscar and Brown, 1985). This method has two main components. The first is to teach the pupils to use certain strategies: ask questions about the text, summarize the text, predict what will happen, and evaluate what has been read. The second component consists of an interactive dialogue between teacher and pupils on the text and the strategies used when processing the text.

The instruction starts with a discussion led by the teacher on what kind of problems a reader can encounter when trying to understand a text. The teacher explains why the four strategies can help. The discussion aims at a metacognitive awareness so that the pupils can steer and supervise their own reading comprehension. The process starts at the sentence or paragraph level, and the teacher shows how the strategies function. When the pupils understand everything, one of them takes over (this is the reciprocal component of the method). The teacher then steers events carefully and gives a feedback to the pupil who is functioning as a teacher. Palinscar and Brown (1985) have carried out several evaluations of this method and found significant improvements in the pupils' reading comprehension.

It is interesting to note that it is in fact possible to help poor readers to develop more effective metacognitive strategies so that they improve their reading comprehension (Rispens, 1990; Spedding and Chan, 1993). This means that it is possible to influence a central aspect of cognitive-intellectual function. This should give teachers, and perhaps particularly special teachers, hope that their job covers more than developing certain skills and knowledge in pupils whose receptivity is not always great. Teaching has a much larger format.

The CRISS programme

Carol M. Santa is the leader of a governmental development project in USA: 'Content Reading Including Study Systems' (CRISS). In this project, she and her colleagues have made a point of precisely developing and conveying methods for helping pupils to develop better reading comprehension (Santa, 1995). One of the main principles in the CRISS project is to recognize that the pupils must be made conscious of their own learning. The thoughts, ideas, and methods are therefore based on giving the pupils an opportunity to take an active part. It is not the teacher's instruction that is most important, but the pupil's learning. The teacher's task is to instruct the pupils how to become good learners, so that they can gradually take more responsibility for - and steering of - their own learning process. While stressing this principle, much emphasis is also put on the teacher's responsibility for showing the pupils how they can think and act in order to gain control of - and be responsible for - their own learning process.

The work related to strengthening the pupils' awareness of their own learning process is developed through conversations, where, at least to start with, the teacher must take the active and leading part. A central idea of the CRISS project is that the teacher is a *model*. He does not only *tell* the pupils what to do - actively and concretely - he demonstrates how they can work, asking searching questions as he progresses (see the paragraph on reciprocal instruction). He then gives the pupils several chances to try out the methods, working in groups as well as individually, and encourages them to talk about what they are doing and why. At the same time as the teacher is demonstrating and allowing the pupils to gain their own experience of the various methods of working, he/she must also show the pupils how to apply the various techniques themselves, and let them see clearly that these techniques can help them to learn. The pupils' awareness is thus steered towards *what* they should learn, and *why* and *how* the various strategies and methods can make it easier for them to reach concrete learning targets. The object is that the pupils should gradually take over the teacher's role.

These are not new and revolutionary ideas. 'Responsibility for own learning' is a well-known slogan. Learning strategies such as word association tasks, explanation of keywords, various note-taking techniques, and drawing pictures on the basis of a text, are strategies that many teachers will recognize. In her book, Santa (1995) situates these study techniques in a theoretical framework which enables us to know not only *what* we must do, but also *why* it is relevant to do it exactly in that manner (see also Broomfield and Combley, 1997; Heaton and Winterston, 1996).

Measures for Children with Writing Difficulties

In most cases of dyslexia, the spelling difficulties are greater than the reading difficulties, and quite often we see that the spelling difficulties persist even though the reading skill gradually improves. Children with writing difficulties tend to have great inhibitions in relation to writing. They thus enter a vicious circle, since they avoid the training necessary to improve their writing skill.

Spelling

Problems with spelling are a typical trait of dyslexia (see Chapter 3). The error pattern may vary somewhat, but we often find many spelling mistakes in connection with irregular words. Why is spelling so problematic for dyslectic pupils? Some researchers think that it is because dyslectics use ineffective spelling strategies (Bråten, 1994). But knowledge of the strategy alone is not enough; metacognitive knowledge and motivation are also required. This is strongly stressed by Bråten, who says that 'in order to be able to use an effective spelling strategy in an independent, reliable, and transferable manner, considerable metacognitive knowledge is also required. This means that the meaning and value of the strategy must be understood in relation to the task to be solved, and that the problem-solving must be controlled or steered in an effective manner. Finally, there must be motivation for attacking the spelling task in a strategic manner' (Bråten, 1994).

Bråten has produced a separate cognitive training programme for poor spellers. It is specially directed at pupils who find it difficult to spell irregular words correctly. Briefly stated, a strategy is explained to the pupils which involves tracing, and the formation of mnemonic rules. Part of the linguistic instructions involve learning that some words are spelt differently than you would think. For example, the following rule might be explicitly taught: '*Island* is spelt *is* + *land*'. Learning this ad hoc 'rule' gives the young speller a verbal correlative to 'hang' the correct spelling on. Other instructions involve verbal memory clues of the type '*Hour* is written with an *h*'. Good results have been obtained with this spelling programme (see Bråten, 1994).

Use of word processing programmes

Data-based word processing programmes may effectively do away with inhibitions related to writing. Since these programmes can check the spelling continuously, the pupil can avoid many frustrations. Immediate corrections also help to drill spelling in effectively. This may have a positive effect on both writing and reading skills.

When dyslectics use word processing programmes, it is important that they do not have to hunt for the letters on the keyboard. Those who have problems with letter recognition, can use keyboards with particularly big letters. In order to benefit properly from word processing programmes, the position of the letters on the keyboard should be learned by heart. This can be done, for example, with the touch method. This gives children a *motor* code for the word which supports the writing process.

Dyslectics may benefit greatly from word processing programmes in tests and exams - provided, of course, that they have learned how to use them. In such situations, it is important that they receive help to correct spelling mistakes. But they should do *all* their work on a computer, because they still need to develop their handwriting, as we are often quite dependent on having functional handwriting. The use of computer should therefore not dominate during the first school years.

Without going into too much detail in respect of the effect of various computer programmes on the market, we would mention that, in general, data technology should play an important role in special education. First of all, the technology can help them tackle their handicap. But there is also a secondary benefit: they become familiar with data technology, and they will profit from this greatly later in life in connection with employment and community life in general. Hands-on experience with computers will probably be of great value in many sectors in life. These techniques may be of particular importance for dyslectics, because they can strengthen their self-confidence considerably.

It often seems to be easier emotionally for many poor writers to be corrected by a computer than by a teacher. Results of research from USA have specially pointed at this fact among adolescents and adults with reading and writing disabilities. The computer does not get tired and discouraged, even when there is not much progress in the development of the pupil's writing, and even when the computer has to correct the same errors again and again. In situations like these, it is easy to understand that human tutors, be they parents or teachers, loose heart from time to time. Poor readers register such signals from their surroundings easily, and emotional inhibitions may thus arise which block the learning process and reduce their self-esteem.

If healthy educational judgement is shown when using the computer, there is little reason to fear adverse effects. Obviously, this tool will only be one of many in order to stimulate and assist the pupils. Children need variation. It is also important to remember that they need human contact. They must not be given the impression that they have been left to themselves with the computer. Human contact is of decisive importance in order to overcome reading and writing difficulties. The computer cannot give the child a hug or stroke its hair - and many pupils who are poor readers need just that.

If the school is to derive maximum benefit from data technology, what is needed most of all is well qualified teachers. They must not only learn how to use the equipment, but also to assess and acquire relevant hardware and software. The market has become so diversified that it is difficult to make a good choice without considerable expertise. Even though the use of data technology may save resources long term, it is important to realize that initially a substantial capital expenditure will be required in order to be able to offer a system of satisfactory quality.

Used in a sensible way, the computer seems to represent a promising tool in the teaching of children and adolescents with reading and writing disabilities (Borgå and Holm, 1993).

Preparing Appropriate Texts for the Dyslexic

To a person with reading difficulties, reading is very hard work. An important task for the teacher is to make the reading easier and thus less of a struggle. For example, the typography can contribute much in this context. In this section, we shall take a closer look at how this can be done.

The *readability* of the text depends on the visual form, whether the layout is well organized, whether the typography is clear, the letters distinct, etc. The linguistic form aims at making the text easy to read. The sentences should be clearly constructed, they should be coherent, the words chosen should not be complicated, and so on. Together, these factors decide the accessibility of the text. The factors interact in a subtle way, and their effect also varies in different groups of readers and fields of reading. The reader's objective also affects the interaction. All these factors make it very difficult to produce general statements about the formulation of texts. New complications arise when modern data technology makes it possible to vary typography, layout, and language in an almost unlimited number of ways. And yet, it may be worth while discussing certain guidelines regarding the forming of the text for dyslexics. In this context, anything that can help reading is worth trying.

Other things being equal, Jansen (1989) states that antiqua-type fonts (like this book is printed with) are easier to read than grotesque-typefaces of the same size - at least in connected text. The reason for this is that letters in antiqua-type fonts have *serifs*, the tiny little 'hooks' at the ends of the line-strokes. (Grotesque typefaces are often called *sans serif*.) The serifs seem to provide a bit more information, and thus help the reader discriminate rapidly between the letters.

What size the letters should have, the line spacing, how long the lines should be, how many lines per page, and the width of margins, are all examples of practical, important questions that research has unfortunately not been able to answer unambiguously.

In general, it is important that the letters making up the word should not be too spread out, so that the word structure is lost (i s l o s t).

The line spacing must be assessed in relation to the height of the letters and the distance between letters and words. Jansen (1989) refers to research and his own experience, and he thinks that line spacing of more than 4.5 mm and less than 2.5 mm may be problematic. Studies of eye movements during the reading process show the importance of quickly finding the beginning of a new line. If the line spacing is not right, this can be more problematic.

As regards line length, it is thought that lines of 45-55 letters seem about right. The size of the book-page and any illustrations are, of course, also of importance when deciding on the optimal solution. When reading, the eye jumps along the line and fixates 5-6 times per line. If the lines are too long, one may get lost; at a minimum, reading becomes too hard. The number of regressions, i.e. when the eye moves back, tends to increase when the lines are much too long.

The more the page in a book is filled with text, the more difficult it is to read. The pages seem to be too compact, and contain so many words that the reader is overwhelmed. The only natural reaction of a person with reading difficulties is to close the book. However, broad margins make the text less compact, and this pleases the reader.

A text should have a straight ('justified') left margin. Paragraphs can be marked by indentations. In research, there is nothing to prove that it is better to leave one line open at the end of every paragraph. On a large page, however, this may make the text seem less compact.

The question of whether the right margin should be straight is not easy to answer. To a poor reader, it might be ideal if one line made up one thought unit. To a writer, such a demand would be very difficult to meet, in fact almost impossible.

With today's desktop programmes, colour printers, and an infinite number of typographic variations, many writers may be tempted to revel in visual effects. From the reader's point of view, and specially the poor reader, this is a nuisance. There is a real need here to stick to essentials.

As mentioned above, one cannot really discuss the visual appearance of a text without being aware of the content and the language to be used. Moreover, one must keep in mind the reader's qualifications. An optimal visual form can probably not make up for content that is not easily accessible and language that feels unnecessarily heavy, but it may make the work easier, and it certainly is not an added burden. In this context, it can be mentioned that many poor, indistinct, and hand-written texts, for example in exams and tests, cause great difficulties for dyslexics.

The Linguistic Formulation of Texts

The linguistic formulation of a text has a decisive effect on how easy or difficult it is to read. All levels of language, from the individual word to larger linguistic structures, help to determine the readability of the text (Santa, 1995).

If the sentences in a text are constructed simply and conventionally, it is easier for the reader to have a general idea what will happen next. Even so, it is rarely possible to know exactly which words will appear. In respect of the content words of a text, (words with a semantic meaning, such as noun, main verb, adjective), it is difficult to predict more than 10% of them in advance (see Gough, 1993). Nonetheless, the context of a simply constructed sentence narrows down the range of what words are possible or likely to appear next.

One factor that can complicate prediction is when a word or phrase comes in front of the *nucleus* of the sentence construction. For example, 'After leaving the party, and after taking the bus home, Roger went to bed'. Here, a lot of material is presented before the main part of the sentence, which is that Roger went to bed. Sentences of this type are usually better broken up into separate thoughts: 'Roger left the party and took the bus home. Then he went to bed.' Another kind of ackward construction are chains of phrases linked by propositions: 'They went to Athens for a week in the summer holidays on a cancellation at half price at very short notice'. Too many phrases containing prepositions appear in a row, and this makes great demands on the reader's short-term memory: When the reader gets to the end of a sentence like this, he or she may well have forgotten what it is all about. The strain on the short-term memory is also obvious when the distance between subject and verb is too great, for example 'Roger, not knowing that his parents weren't coming home that evening, wondered why the house was so empty.' We know that dyslexics often have a poor short-term memory for words. Thus, they find such clumsy constructions particularly difficult to cope with.

Beck et al. (1984) have shown that if a text is revised and simplified on the basis of educational principles, it will become considerably more accessible to poor readers. When they removed formulations that they thought might cause problems, the readers understood the text better, and remembered more of the important concepts from such texts than from texts that were not specially adapted.

Elbro (1989b) has described in detail several examples of what revision of texts on the basis of educational principles can lead to. He has demonstrated how a revised text often contains tightly compressed information, and therefore becomes slightly longer than it was. Revision should also lead to more normalized language and the use of more words and expressions of high frequency. Compound words should often be split up, so that rarely used words like *fjord ice* are replaced by the more common expression, *ice on the fjord.* This normalization also means that the words in the revised version are used in their normal sense. No simplification of content is necessarily required. On the whole, the reader gets the same information in the revised text.

In a so-called field analysis, Elbro shows how syntactic simplification can be carried out through revision based on educational principles. In order for the reader to get the text to cohere, he/she has to add something of his/her own knowledge of the world. In the example: 'Lisa came tumbling down the stairs. Robert went off to get hold of a doctor', it is clear to the reader that Lisa hurt herself when she fell on the stairs. Yet this fact appears nowhere in the text. The reader understands this by reading between the lines. He goes beyond the information that has been given.

The following example is easily understood by a child from the Western culture: 'Sara was going to a party. She was wondering if Elin would like to get a book. She shook the piggy bank. Not a sound was heard.' A child from another culture might be rather confused. The assertion in one sentence is not linked up with that in the following sentence. There is no framework in which to place the various assertions. Without knowledge of what takes place in childrens' parties, it is quite impossible - after the first assertion - to understand that 'she' (whoever that may be) is wondering whether Elin likes a certain book, etc. The problem here for a child from another culture is not linguistic; the sentences are clear and crisp. The problem is that the semantic putty that binds the sentences together is lacking in the child's repertoire of cultural knowledge.

A text can also be clarified by introducing linguistic ties to hold the text together. Such ties can be conjunctions, unambiguous pronouns, repetition of key words, etc.

A text revision must, of course, be aimed at a possible target group. For very poor readers, who still have problems with decoding words, the length and frequency of words must be considered, the type of orthographic structure they are given, and to the extent to which they are concrete and clear. If the readers are more advanced, the over-all construction of the text should be focused specially upon.

Choice of Reading Texts for the Dyslexic

It should by now be apparent that good revision of a text is not a mechanical procedure, based on any simple formula. Even so, the quest for a reliable formula has had a strange attraction. To many, the ideal has been to be able to run a text on a computer, and have it simplified and structured so that it is better suited for a certain target group, for example poor readers.

For a long time, attempts have been made to develop a method for measuring the difficulty of texts. This could then be used to select suitable texts, and as an aid to writers, so that the texts would be easier to read. One attempt at formulating such a formula is Björnsson concept of 'lix' (Björnsson, 1968).

'Lix' is based on the observation that sentence length and word length are two factors which give us an indication as to the many-sided nature of grammar and difficulties with words. The formula is Lix = Lm + Lo, where Lm is the average number of words in each sentence, and Lo the percentage of long words (more than 6 letters). Lix-values of 10-20 are considered to be very easy texts, while values of up to 60 indicate very difficult texts.

However, the formula only measures the external properties of the text and does not take into account how strange or familiar the content is, or how the ideas are structured. It is simple to use, and this may be why it is so popular. Elbro (1989b) has shown that, with very simple means, texts can be adapted so that they get a low lix-value, but that they do not necessarily become easier to read.

Information density cannot be measured by means of lix. Perfetti (1969) has tried to construct a method for measuring the difficulty of a text by estimating the relationship between the content words and all the words in a text. The problem connected with this type of formal attempt is that one cannot really characterize a text without considering the reader. Joseph Conrad once wrote to a friend: 'As an author, I really only write half the book; the reader does the rest'. The meaning is not in the book, nor is it in the reader's head, but it is created in a field of tension between each individual reader and the text.

One important measure for assessing how useful a text is, is the extent to which it invites discussions and collaboration (see earlier discussion on the social dimension of reading). Acquisition of knowledge is largely a social dimension. Lix naturally tells us nothing about this. Altogether, lix says little about how easily available a text is.

Emphasizing Strong Sides of Dyslexics

It is important to remember that the cognitive style and cognitive qualifications of many dyslexics may in fact have some advantages. West (1992) has demonstrated that many dyslexics may have particularly strong visual and spatial abilities, and this may be why some of them have special abilities in mathematics, science, technical subjects, and data sciences. It is well known that many eminent scientists and technicians have or have had clear dyslexic problems. Many dyslexics distinguish themselves in subjects that demand creativity and new ideas.

Modern information technology has visual and graphic aspects that give those with well-developed abilities at perceiving patterns and three-dimensional figures an obvious advantage. Dyslexics with this ability can thus make a constructive and important contribution to information technology, often specially because they are able to alter design and information in a creative manner (West, 1992).

Many dyslexics also have a good memory for colours and are able to make use of all their senses for learning and solving problems. Instead of verbal descriptions, they can see patterns with their inner eye. In conventional and verbal-oriented training and in social situations needing written language skills, the dyslexic does not show to advantage. On the other hand, an important challenge to society is to make use of the special resources that many dyslexics have in other fields. There is reason to believe that society has an unused human capital here, which should not be wasted.

In the USA, good results have also been obtained by using music and rhythm in the reading instruction of poor readers (Douglas and Willatts, 1994; Lamb and Gregory, 1993). In general, it is important to have knowledge of the strong sides of dyslexics and make use of these to compensate for reading and writing problems.

But the object is not only to make them skilful readers, but also to make them love reading. The latter is a challenging task for the teacher. In the book 'Fostering the Love of Reading' (Cramer and Castle, 1994), much good advice is given on what home and school can do to achieve this objective.

Alternative Methods

A number of *alternative methods* for treating dyslexics have appeared in recent years. A characteristic of these is that they promise a rapid and reliable solution of the dyslexia problem. The reason for this development may be that the traditional methods of treatment are considered by some to be time-consuming and not very effective.

It is understandable in many ways that parents look for alternative methods when their children are struggling with great reading problems, and traditional remediation has not given the hoped-for result. Who would not do everything possible to help her own children? Under these circumstances, one cannot expect critical questions to be asked about the scientific validity of the method. Teachers have also experienced some uncertainty as to which attitude they should adopt to these alternative methods of treatment. Should one perhaps be more open and positive to these new ideas? Can the alternative forms of treatment help pupils with great reading problems?

Over the years, radical and sometimes drastic treatment procedures have been suggested. However, these have not been properly tried out, and they are often based on speculative theories (for a review see Allington and Walmsley, 1996; Spafford and Grosser, 1996). Some might maintain that the main thing is that the remediation works in practice, regardless of whether or not it has any scientific support. However, we consider that this type of attitude unacceptable. A justifiable treatment programme should be based on experience and scientific control. It is possible that the positive effects sometimes observed with alternative methods of treatment are the result of the extra attention given to the pupil during the use of the method. American doctors have a saying: 'You should treat as many patients as possible with the new drug as long as it is still has the power to heal'. In medicine, the placebo effect is a well-known phenomenon. However, neither doctors nor special teachers should rely on the placebo effect for ever. We must look for methods that are theoretically understandable, and that have been subjected to systematic trials using tested methods. Without insight and comprehension, teaching becomes an empty shell in the long run.

Prognosis for Pupils with Dyslexia

The positive message is that the great majority of pupils can learn to read if they are early-on given a well-tailored instruction programme. This has been shown in a recent investigation by Vellutino et al. (1996).

At the start of the first grade, the pupils who showed problems in learning to read, and also had phonological problems, were selected. About 15% of the whole pupil group were classified as being at risk. These were offered intensive instruction, and one-to-one tuition. The instruction included an emphasis on training both phonological skills and reading (explicit training in word decoding, as well as much reading of appropriate reading texts). By the end of the first grade, most of the pupils had a reading skill corresponding to their age. But there was a small group, 1.5 percent of the total group, who, in spite of the intensive instruction, had made little or no progress either in phonological skills or in reading. As regards these pupils, it must be asked whether they would have been better helped with a reading method that made less demands on phonological skills.

But the encouraging aspect of Vellutino's investigation is that early and systematic help to pupils at risk gives good results. This is in accord with research results by Naylor et al. (1990). In a follow-up of 87 dyslexics over a period of 20 years, they showed that early diagnosis and early supportive measures could give a third of the pupils a normal reading function. But even so, only 19 percent were able to master their spelling problems.

But on the other hand, some research has shown that dyslexia persists in some individuals right up to adulthood (for example Bruck, 1990; Fowler and Scarborough, 1993; White, 1992). As we have seen, the problems appear specially when they read new words and nonwords. Jacobson and Lundberg (forthcoming) followed up 92 pupils with poor reading skill in the 2nd grade. Most of them still had reading problems in the 9th grade. These results agree with those reported by many researchers on the reading development in poor readers (for review see Kavale and Reese, 1992).

The serious question is: what are the consequences of this handicap for these people? Reiff et al. (1994) carried out extensive and detailed interviews of 71 adult dyslexics who had had success in life both professionally and financially. Common to all of there 'successful' dyslexics was that they had to struggle to gain control over their lives, they were goal-oriented, and had a burning desire to succeed in life. They had obviously succeeded in breaking through the passivity, resignation, and learnt helplessness which are so typical of those who have trouble in learning because of reading problems. There is reason to believe that good social support and guidance can lead to active adaptation strategies. But we still know too little about the factors that determine which individual dyslexics achieve a good life quality despite their serious functional handicap. We need to know more about the extent to which the following factors affect reading development: access to support, educational resources, cognitive learning style, level of stress, different personalities, and lifestyle. In brief, we need extended research on dyslexia.

Conclusion and Comments

Every individual pupil is special. It is therefore not possible to give an outline of a programme that is suitable for poor readers in general. We have previously pointed out some factors that, generally speaking, promote reading and writing learning, but in addition there are measures that only become advisable after a thorough assessment of the individual pupil's decoding and comprehension processes.

In any case, it is important that the assessment is a continuous process, so that one always knows how the instruction programme is functioning. If the recommended programme is not giving the desired result, it is necessary to make new investigations and to adjust the educational programme.

We all need to succeed in what we are doing. Success is the key to teaching pupils with reading and writing problems. We cannot expect poor readers to exert themselves unduly if they have experienced that earlier efforts have been of little benefit. Here, we will present what we would like to call a cost-benefit model, which applies generally, and particularly to pupils with reading and writing problems.

The challenge to the teacher is to find an instruction programme that gives a correct balance between costs and benefits. The programme must not be too easy, because then the pupil does not find it exciting and challenging. On the other hand, it must not be too difficult, because then the benefit will be felt to be poor compared with the efforts exerted by the pupil. In order to find the correct balance, it is essential that the teacher has good knowledge of the individual pupil's interests and learning capacity.

Brief Summary

At the beginning of this chapter, we first directed attention to various problems connected with the evaluation of the remediation, and then we gave an account of some general principles of the teacher's work. Here, we emphasize the importance of overlearning and automatization in the learning process.

We then mentioned a very important component of the special education of dyslexic pupils: exercises in phonological awareness. Recent research has clearly documented the benefit of such exercises. Our description includes use of multisensory stimulation, the books with cassette tapes, and computers in the instruction of dyslexics. Finally we gave an account of some measure which promote reading comprehension, and we reflected on the long-term prognosis for dyslexic pupils.

REFERENCES

Aaron, P. (1989). Can reading disabilities be diagnosed without using intelligence tests? *Journal of Learning Disabilities, 24,* 178-186.

Aaron, P. (1997). The impending demise of the discrepancy formula. *Review of Educational Research, 67,* 461-502.

Aasved, H. (1988). Visual-ocular control of normal and learning-disabled children. *Developmental Medical Child Neurologica, 29,* 477-487.

Ackerman, P. (1994). EEG power spectra of children with dyslexia, slow learners, and normally reading children with ADD during verbal processing. *Journal of Learning Disabilities, 27,* 619-630.

Adams, M. (1990). *Beginning to read.* Cambridge, Mass.: MIT Press.

Adams, M., Foorman, B., Lundberg, I., & Beeler, T. (1998). *Phonemic awareness in young children.* Baltimore, MD: Paul Brookes.

Allington, R., & Walmsley, S. (1996). *No quick fix: Rethinking literacy programs in American elementary schools.* Newark, DE: International Reading Association.

Alm, J., & Andersson, J. (1995). *Läs- och skrivsvårigheter på kriminalvårdsanstalter i Uppsala län.* Uppsala: AMI.

Annell, A., Gustavson, H., & Tenstam, J. (1970). Symptomology in school boys with positive sex Chromatin (the Klinefelter's syndrome). *Acta Psychiatrica Scandinavica, 46,* 71-80.

Backman, J., Bruck, M., Hiebert, M., & Seidenberg, M. (1984). Acquisition and use of spelling sound correspondences in reading. *Journal of Experimental Child Psychology, 38,* 114-133.

Baddeley, A. (1986). *Working memory.* Oxford: Oxford University Press.

Badian, N. (1994). Do dyslexic and other poor readers differ in reading-related cognitive skills? *Reading and Writing: An Interdisciplinary Journal, 6,* 45-63.

Badian, N. (1997). Dyslexia and the double deficit hypothesis. *Annals of Dyslexia, 47,* 69-88.

Bailet, L. (1990). Spelling rule usage among students with learning disabilities and normally achieving students. *Journal of Learning Disabilities, 23,* 121-128.

Baker, L., Afflerbach, P., & Reinking, D. (Eds). (1996). *Developing engaged in school and home communities.* Mahwah, NJ: Lawrence Erlbaum Associates.

Ball, E., & Blachman, B. (1988). Phoneme segmentation training: Effect on reading readiness. *Annals of Dyslexia, 38,* 208-225.

Ball, E., & Blachman, B. (1991). Does phoneme awareness training in kindergarten make a difference in early word recognition and developmental spelling? *Reading Research Quarterly, 26,* 49-66.

Beauvois, M., & Derouesné, J. (1981). Lexical or ortographic agraphia. *Brain, 104,* 21-49.

Beck, I., McKeown, M., Omanson, R., & Pople, M. (1984). Improving the comprehensibility of stories. The effect of revisions that improve coherence. *Reading Research Quarterly, 19,* 252-257.

Berlin, R. (1887). *Eine besondere Art von Wortblindheit (Dyslexie).* Wiesbaden: Verlag von J. F. Bergmann.

Berninger, V. (Ed.) (1994). *The varieties of orthographic knowledge. I: Theoretical and developmental issues* London: Kluwer Academic Publishers.

Berninger, V. (Ed.) (1995). *The varieties of orthographic knowledge, II: Relationship to phonology, reading and writing.* London: Kluwer Academic Publishers.

Berninger, V. (1996). *Reading and writing acquisition. A developmental neuropsychological perspective.* Boulder, CO: Westview Press.

Berninger, V. (1997). Educational and biological links to learning disabilities. *Perspectives. The International Dyslexia Association, 23,* 10-13.

Berninger, V., & Abbot, R. (1994). Redefining learning disabilities: Moving beyond aptitude-achievement discrepancies to failure to respond to valid treatment protocols. In G. Lyon (Ed.), *Frames of references for the assessment of learning disabilities* Baltimore, MD: Paul Brookes.

Bishop, D. (1989). Unstable vergence control and dyslexia - a critique. *British Journal of Ophthalmology, 73,* 223-245.

Björnsson, C. (1968). *Läsbarhet.* Stockholm: Almquist & Wiksell.

Bjaalid, I.-K., & Høien., T. (1996). Diagnosing word recognition problems: A process-analytic approach. *Nordisk Tidsskrift for Spesialpedagogikk, 2,* 42-50.

Bjaalid, I.-K., Høien, T., & Lundberg, I. (1993). Letter identification and lateral masking in dyslexics and normal readers. *Scandinavian Journal of Educational Research, 37,* 151-161.

Bjaalid, I.-K., Høien, T., & Lundberg, I. (1995). A comparison of components in word recognition between dyslexic and normal readers. *Scandinavian Journal of Educational Research, 29,* 51-59.

Bjaalid, I.-K., Høien, T., & Lundberg, I. (1996). The contribution of orthographic and phonological processes to word reading in young Norwegian readers. *Reading and Writing: An Interdisciplinary Journal, 8,* 189-198.

Bjaalid, I.-K., Høien, T., & Lundberg, I. (1997). Dual-route and connectionist models: A step towards a combined model. *Scandinavian Journal of Psychology, 37,* 73-82.

Blachman, B. (1984). Relationship of rapid naming ability and language analysis skills to kindergarten and first-grade reading achievement. *Journal of Educational Psychology, 76,* 610-622.

Blachman, B. (1997). Early intervention and phonological awareness: A cautionary tale. In B. Blachman (Ed.), *Foundations of reading acquisition and dyslexia. Implications for early intervention.* London: Lawrence Erlbaum Associates.

Boder, E. (1971). Developmental dyslexia: Prevailing diagnostic concepts and a new diagnostic approach. In H. Myklebust (Ed.), *Progress in learning disabilities.* New York: Grune & Stratton.

Boder, E. (1973). Developmental dyslexia: A diagnostic screening procedure based on three characteristic patterns of reading and spelling. In B. Bateman (Ed.), *Learning disorders.* Seattle: Special Child Publication.

Boder, E., & Jarrico, S. (1984). A diagnostic screening test for subtypes of dyslexia: The Boder test of reading-spelling patterns. In R. Malatesha & H. Whitaker (Eds.), *Dyslexia: A global issue.* Haag: Martinus Nijhoff.

Borgå, M., & Holm, M. (1993). *EDB i spesialundervisning.* Oslo: Ad Notam Gyldendal.

Borström, I., & Elbro, C. (1997). Prevention of dyslexia in kindergarten: Effects of phonological awareness training. In C. Hulme & M. Snowling (Eds.), *Dyslexia: Biology, cognition, and intervention.* London: Whurr.

Bradley, L. (1981). A tactile approach to reading. *Special Education: Forward Trends, 8,* 32-36.

Bradley, L., & Bryant, P. (1985). *Rhyme and reason in reading and spelling* [I.A.R.L.D. Monographs No 1]. Ann Arbor: University of Michigan Press.

Brady, S. (1997). Abilities to encode phonological representations: An underlying difficulty of poor readers. In B. Blachman (Ed.), *Foundations of reading acquisition and dyslexia. Implications for early intervention.* London: Lawrence Erlbaum Associates.

Brady, S., & Shankweiler, D. (1991). *Phonological processes in literacy.* Hillsdale, NJ: Lawrence Erlbaum Associates.

Bransford, J., Stein, B., & Vye, N. (1982). Helping students learn how to learn from written texts. In M. Singer (Ed.), *Competent reader, disabled reader: Research and application.* Hillsdale, NJ: Erlbaum.

Breitmeyer, B. (1993). Sustained (P) and Transient (M) channels in vision: A review and implications for reading. In D. Willows, R. Kruk, & E. Corcos (Eds.), *Visual processes in reading and reading disabilities.* Hillsdale, NJ: Lawrence Erlbaum Associates.

Broomfield, H., & Combley, M. (1997). *Overcoming dyslexia: A practical handbook for the classroom.* London: Whurr.

Bruck, M. (1988). The word recognition and spelling of dyslexic children. *Reading Research Quarterly, 23,* 51-69.

Bruck, M. (1990). Word recognition skills of adults with childhood diagnoses of dyslexia. *Developmental Psychology, 26,* 439-454.

Bruck, M. (1992). Persistence of dyslexics' phonological awareness deficits. *Developmental Psychology, 28,* 874-886.

Bruck, M. (1998). Outcomes of adults with childhood histories of dyslexia. In C. Hulme & M. Joshi (Eds.), *Reading and spelling. Development and disorders*. Mahwah, NJ: Lawrence Erlbaum Associates.

Bruck, M., & Treiman, R. (1990). Phonological awareness and spelling in normal children and dyslexics: The case of initial consonant clusters. *Journal of Experimental Child Psychology, 50*, 90-108.

Bryant, P., & Bradley, L. (1980). Why children sometimes write words they cannot read. In U. Frith (Ed.), *Cognitive processes in spelling*. London: Academic Press.

Bryant, P., & Bradley, L. (1985). *Children's reading problems*. Oxford: Blackwell.

Bryant, P., & Impey, L. (1986). The similarities between normal readers and developmental and acquired dyslexics. *Cognition, 24*, 121-137.

Bryant, P., Bradley, L., McLean, M., & Crossland, J. (1989). Nursery ryhmes, phonological skills and reading. *Journal of Child Language, 16*, 407-428.

Bråten, I. (1990). *Kognitive strategier og ortografi*. Oslo: Pedagogisk Forskningsinstitutt, Universitetet i Oslo (doctoral thesis).

Bråten, I. (1994). *Learning to spell. Training orthographic problem-solving with poor spellers: A strategy instructional approach*. Oslo: Scandinavian University Press.

Byrne, B., & Fielding-Barnsley, R. (1993). Evaluation of a program to teach phonemic awareness to young children: A 1-year follow-up. *Journal of Educational Psychology, 85*, 104-111.

Byrne, B., & Fielding-Barnsley, R. (1995). Evaluation of a program to teach phonemic awareness to young children: A 2 and 3-year follow-up and a new preschool trial. *Journal of Educational Psychology, 85*, 1-5.

Cain, K. (1996). Story knowledge and comprehension skill. In C. Cornoldi & J. Oakhill (Eds.), *Reading comprehension difficulties. Processes and intervention*. Mahwah, NJ: Lawrence Erlbaum Associates.

Cain, K., & Oakhill, J. (1998). Comprehension, skill and inference-making ability: Issues of causality. In C. Hulme & M. Joshi (Eds.), *Reading and spelling. Development and disorders*. Mahwah, NJ: Lawrence Erlbaum Associates.

Cain, K., & Oakhill, J. (1999). Inference making ability and its relation to comprehension failure in young children. *Reading and Writing: An Interdisciplinary Journal, 11*, 489-503.

Cardon, L., Smith, S., Fulker, D., Kimberling, W., Pennington, B., & DeFries, J. (1994). Quantitative trait locus for reading disability on chromosome 6. *Science, 266*, 276-279.

Carr, S., & Thompson, B. (1996). The effects of prior knowledge and schema activation strategies on the inferential reading comprehension of children with and without learning disabilities. *Learning Disability Quarterly, 19*, 48-61.

Castle, A., & Coltheart, M. (1993). Varieties of developmental dyslexia. *Cognition, 47*, 141-151.

Center, Y., Wheldall, K., Freeman, L., Outhred, L., & McNaught, M. (1995). Evaluation of Reading Research. *Reading Research Quarterly, 30*, 240-263.

Chall, J. (1983). *Stages of reading development*. New York: McGraw-Hill.

Chapman, Y., & Tunmer, W. (1993). Recovering Reading Recovery. *Australia and New Zealand Journal of Developmental Disabilities, 17*, 59-71.

Chomsky, C. (1970). Phonology and reading. In H. Levin & J. Williams (Eds.), *Basic studies in reading*. New York: Basic Books.

Cicci, R. (1983). Disorders of written language. In H. Myklebust (Ed.), *Progress in learning disabilities*. New York: Grune & Stratton.

Clay, M. (1985). *The early detection of complex behavior*. Auckland, New Zealand: Heinemann.

Coltheart, M., Patterson, K., & Marshall, J. (1980). *Deep dyslexia*. London: Routledge & Kegan Paul.

Courchesne, E., & Plante, E. (1997). Measurement and analysis issues in neurodevelopmental magnetic resonance imaging. In R. Tatcher (Ed.), *Developmental neuroimaging: Mapping the development of brain and behaviour*. London: Academic Press.

Craig, M., & Yore, L. (1996). Middle school student's awareness of strategies for resolving comprehension difficulties in science reading. *Journal of Research and Development in Reading, 29*, 226-238.

Crain, S., & Shankweiler, D. (1990). Explaining failures in spoken language comprehension by children with reading disability. In D. Balota, G. Flores d'Arcais, & K. Rayner (Eds.), *Comprehension processes in reading*. Hillsdale, NJ: Lawrence Erlbaum Associates.

Cramer, E., & Castle, M. (1994). *Fostering the love of reading: The affective domain*. Newark, DE: International Reading Association.

Critchley, M. (1970). *Aphasiology and other aspects of language*. London: Edward Arnold.

Davidson, R., & Hugdahl, K. (1995). *Brain asymmetry.* Cambridge, Mass: MIT Press.

Decker, S., & Vandenberg, S. (1985). Converging evidence for multiple genetic forms of reading disability. *Brain and Language, 33,* 197-215.

DeFries, J., Alarcon, M., & Olson, R. (1997). Genetic aetiologies of reading and spelling deficits. Brain, mind, and behaviour in dyslexia. In C. Hulme & M. Snowling (Eds.), *Dyslexia: Biology, cognition, and intervention*. London: Whurr.

DeFries, J., Stevenson, J., Gillis, J., & Wadsworth, S. (1991). Genetic etiology of spelling deficits in the Colorado and London twin studies of reading disabilities. In B. Pennington (Ed.), *Reading disabilities: Genetic and neurological influences*. London: Kluwer Academic Publishers.

DeFries, J., Vogel, G., & LaBuda, M. (1985). Colorado family reading study: An overview. In J. Fuller & E. Simmel (Eds.), *Behavioral genetics: Principles and applications, II*. Hillsdale, N.J.: Lawrence Erlbaum Associates .

Desberg, P., Elliot, D., & Marsh, G. (1980). American black English and spelling. In U. Frith (Ed.), *Cognitive processes in spelling*. London: Academic Press.

Dougherty, K., & Johnston, J. (1996). Overlearning, fluency, and automaticity. *Behavior Analyst, 19,* 289-293.

Douglas, S., & Willatts, P. (1994). The relationship between musical ability and literacy skills. *Journal of Research in Reading, 17,* 99-107.

Dowhower, S. (1994). Repeated reading revisited: Research into practice. *Reading and Writing Quarterly: Overcoming Learning Difficulties, 10,* 343-358.

Downing, J. (1979). *Reading and reasoning* . New York: Springer-Verlag.

Duane, D. (1999). *Reading and attention disorders. Neurobiological correlates*. Timonium, MD: York Press.

Duane, D., & Gray, D. (1991). *The Reading Brain. The Biological Basis of Dyslexia*. Parkton, MD: York Press.

Duffy, F. (1989). Brain Electrical Activity Mapping (BEAM) in dyslexia. The Rodin Remediation Academy Conference. Dublin.

Dunlop, P. (1972). Dyslexia: The orthoptic approach. *Australian Journal of Orthoptics, 12,* 16-20.

Durkin, D. (1978-1979). What classroom observations reveal about reading comprehension instruction. *Reading Research Quarterly, 14,* 481-533.

Ehri, L. (1991). Development of the ability to read words. In R. Barr, M. Kamil, & P. Mosenthal (Eds.), *Handbook of reading research, Vol. 2* New York: Longman.

Ehri, L. (1992). Reconceptualizing the development of sight word reading and its relationship to recoding. In P. Gough, L. Ehri, & R. Treiman (Eds.), *Reading acquisition*. Hillsdale, NJ: Erlbaum.

Ehri, L., & Wilce, L. (1985). Movement into reading: Is the first stage of printed word learning visual or phonetic? *Reading Research Quarterly, 20,* 163-179.

Elbro, C. (1989a). Morphological awareness in dyslexia. In C. von Euler, I. Lundberg, & G. Lennerstrand (Eds.), *Brain and Reading*. London: MacMillan.

Elbro, C. (1989b) Teksters sproglige tilgængelighed. In M. Dalby, C. Elbro, M. Jansen, & T. Krogh (Eds.), *Bogen om Læsning II*. København: Munksgaard.

Elbro, C. (1990). *Differences in dyslexia*. Copenhagen: Munksgaard.

Elbro, C. (1996). Early linguistic abilities and reading development: A review and a hypothesis. *Reading and Writing: An Interdisciplinary Journal, 8,* 453-485.

Elbro, C. (1997). Reading-listening discrepancy definitions of dyslexia. In R. Reitsma & L. Verhoeven (Eds.), *Problems and interventions in literacy development*. Dordrecht: Vrie Universitet.

Elbro, C., & Arnbak, E. (1996). The role of morpheme recognition and morphological awareness in dyslexia. *Annals of Dyslexia, 46, 209-240.*

Elbro, C., Nielsen, I., & Petersen, D. (1994). Dyslexia in adults: Evidence for deficits in non-word reading and in the phonological representation of lexical items. *Annals of Dyslexia, 54,* 205-226.

Elbro, C., Petersen, D., & Borstrøm, I. (1998). Prediciting dyslexia from kindergarten. The importance of distinctness of phonological representations of lexical items. *Reading Research Quarterly, 33*, 36-60.

Elkonin, D. (1973). U.S.S.R. In J. Downing (Ed.), *Comparative reading*. New York: MacMillan.

Elley, W. (1994). *The IEA study of reading literacy: Achievement and instruction in thirty-two school systems* Exeter: Pergamon.

Engen, L. (1996). *Tidlig hjelp. En praktisk, metodisk beskrivelse av et treningsopplegg for lesesvake elever i 1. og 2. klasse.* Stavanger: Senter for leseforsking.

Fawcett, A., & Nicolson, R. (1993). Speed of processing, motor skill, automaticity and dyslexia. In A. Fawcett & R. Nicolson (Eds.), *Dyslexia in Children: Multidisciplinary Perspectives* London: Harvester Wheatsheaf.

Fawcett, A., & Nicolson, R. (1994). Dyslexia: Evidence for deficits in non-word reading and in the phonological representation of lexical items. *Annals of Dyslexia, 54*, 204-226.

Felton, R., Naylor, C., & Wood, F. (1990). Neuropsychological profile of adult dyslexics. *Brain and Language, 39*, 485-497.

Fernald, G. (1943). *Remedial techniques in basic school subjects*. New York: McGraw-Hill.

Fletcher, J., & Foorman, B. (1994). Issues in definition and measurement of learning disabilities: The need for early intervention. In G. Lyon (Ed.), *Frames of references for the assessment of learning disabilities*. Baltimore: Paul Brookes.

Fletcher, J., & Morris, D. (1997). Subtypes of dyslexia: An old problem revisited. In B. Blachman (Ed.), *Foundations of reading acquisition and dyslexia*. London: Lawrence Erlbaum Associates.

Foorman, B., Francis, D., Shaywitz, S., Shaywitz, B., & Fletcher, J. (1997). The case of early reading intervention. In B. Blachman (Ed.), *Foundations of reading acquisition and dyslexia. Implications for early intervention*. London: Lawrence Erlbaum Associates.

Fowler, R., & Scarborough, H. (1993). *Should reading disabled adults be distuinguished from other adults seeking literacy instruction? A review of theory and research*. New Haven: Unpublished.

Francis, D., Shaywitz, S., Stuebing, K., Shaywitz, B., & Fletcher, J. (1994). Measurement of change: Assessing behavior over time and within a developmental context. In G. Lyon (Ed.), *Frames of reference for the assessment of learning disabilities. New views on measurement issues*. Baltimore, Maryland: Paul Brookes.

Francis, D., Shaywitz, S., Stuebing, K., Shaywitz, B., & Fletcher, J. (1996). Developmental lag versus deficit models of reading disability: A longitudinal growth curves analysis. *Journal of Educational Psychology, 88*, 3-17.

Frith, U. (1980). Unexpected spelling problems. In U. Frith (Ed.), *Cognitive processes in spelling*. London: Academic Press.

Frith, U. (1985). Beneath the surface of developmental dyslexia. In K. Patterson, J. Marshall, & M. Coltheart (Eds.), *Surface dyslexia*. London: Lawrence Erlbaum Associates.

Frith, U. (1997). Brain, mind, and behaviour in dyslexia. In C. Hulme & M. Snowling (Eds.), *Dyslexia: Biology, cognition, and intervention* London: Whurr.

Galaburda, A. (1993). *Dyslexia and development. Neurobiological aspects of extra-ordinary brains.* Cambridge, MA: Harvard University Press.

Galaburda, A., & Kemper, T. (1979). Cytoarchitectonic abnormalities in developmental dyslexia: A case study. *Annals of Dyslexia, 6*, 94-100.

Galaburda, A., Aboitiz, F., Rosen, G., & Sherman, G. (1985). Histological asymmetry in the primary visual cortex of the rat: Implications for mechanisms of cerebral asymmetry. *Cortex, 22*, 151-160.

Galaburda, A., Corsiglia, J., Rosen, G., et al. (1987). Planum temporale asymmetry, reappraisal since Geschwind and Levitsky. *Neuropsychologia, 25*, 853-868.

Galaburda, A., Menard, M., & Rosen, G. (1994). Evidence for aberrant auditory anatomy in developmental dyslexia. *Proceedings of the National Academy of Sciences, 91*, 8010-8013.

Galaburda, A., Rosen, G., & Sherman, G. (1989). The neural origin of developmental dyslexia: Implications for medicine, neurology and cognition. In A. Galaburda (Ed.), *From reading to neurons*. Cambridge, MA: MIT Press.

Gallagher, A., Laxon, V., Armstrong, E., & Frith, U. (1996). Phonological difficulties in high functioning dyslexics. *Reading and Writing: An Interdisciplinary Journal, 8,* 499-509.

Geiger, G., & Lettvin, J. (1987). Peripheral vision in persons with dyslexia. *New England Journal of Medicine, 316,* 1238-1243.

Geschwind, N. (1985). Dyslexia in neurological perspective. In F. Duffy & N. Geschwind (Eds.), *Dyslexia. A neuroscientific approach to clinical evaluation.* Boston: Little, Brown and Company.

Geschwind, N., & Behan, P. (1982). Lefthandedness: Association with immune disease, migrain, and developmental learning disorder. In *Proceeding of the National Academy of Sciences.* National Academy of Sciences.

Geschwind, N., & Behan, P. (1984). Laterality, hormones and immunity. In N. Geschwind & A. Galaburda (Eds.), *Cerebral dominance: The biological foundations.* Cambridge, Mass.: Harvard University Press.

Geschwind, N., & Galaburda, A. (1984). *Cerebral dominance: The biological foundations.* Cambridge, Mass.: Harvard University Press.

Geschwind, N., & Levitsky, W. (1968). Human brain: Left – right asymmetries in temporal speech region. *Science, 161,* 186-187.

Gjessing, H. (1977). *Dysleksi.* Oslo: Universitetsforlaget.

Glezheiser, L., & Clark, D. (1991). Early reading and instruction. In B. Wong (Ed.), *Learning about strategies.* San Diego, CA: Academic Press.

Glushko, R. (1979). The organization and activation of orthographic knowledge in reading aloud. *Journal of Experimental Psychology: Human Perception and Performance, 5,* 674-691.

Goldblum, N., & Frost, R. (1988). The crossword puzzle paradigm: The effectiveness of different word fragments as cues for the retrieval of words. *Memory and Cognition, 16,* 158-166.

Goodman, K. (1976). A psycholinguistic guessing game. In H. Singer & R. Ruddell (Eds.), *Theoretical models and processes of reading.* Newark: Del.: International Reading Association.

Goswami, U. (1994). Reading by analogy: Theoretical and practical perspectives. In C. Hulme & M. Snowling (Eds.), *Reading development and dyslexia* London: Whurr.

Goswami, U. (1997). Learning to read different orthographies: Phonological awareness, orthographic representations and dyslexia. In C. Hulme & M. Snowling (Eds.), *Dyslexia: Biology, cognition, and intervention.* London: Whurr.

Goswami, U., & Bryant, P. (1990). *Phonological skills and learning to read.* Hillsdale, NJ: Lawrence Erlbaum Associates.

Goswami, U., & Mead, F. (1992). Onset and rime awareness and analogies in reading. *Reading Research Quarterly, 27,* 152-162.

Gough, P. (1993). The beginning of reading. *Reading and Writing: An Interdisciplinary Journal, 5,* 181-192.

Gough, P., & Hillinger, M. (1980). Learning to read: An unnatural act. *Bulletin of the Orton Society, 30,* 171-176.

Gough, P., & Tunmer, W. (1986). Decoding, reading, and reading disability. *Remedial and Special Education, 7,* 6-10.

Grigorenko, E. (1997). Linkage analyses on Chromosomes 1, 6 and 15. In G. Pavlidis (Ed.), *Abstracts.* 4th World Congress on Dyslexia. Macedonia, Greece.

Gross-Glenn, K., Jallad, B., Novoa, L., Helgren-Lempesis, V., & Lubs, H. (1990). Nonsense passage reading as a diagnostic aid in the study of adult familial dyslexia. *Reading and Writing: An Interdisciplinary Journal, 2,* 161-173.

Guthrie, J., & Wigfield, A. (1997). *Reading engagement. Motivating readers through integrated instruction.* Newark, DE: International Reading Association.

Hall, S., & Moats, L. (1999). *Straight talk about reading.* Chicago, Ill.: Contemporary Books.

Hansen, J., & Pearson, P. (1983). An instructional study: Improving the inferential comprehension of good and poor fourthgrade readers. *Journal of Educational Psychology, 75,* 221-229.

Harris, P., & Sipay, E. (1985). *How to increase reading ability.* New York: Longman.

Harris, P., Kruithof, A., Terwogt, M., & Visser, T. (1981). Children's detection and awareness of textual anomaly. *Journal of Experimental Child Psychology, 31,* 212-230.

Hayes, J., & Flower, L. (1980). Identifying the organization of writing processes. In L. Gregg & E. Steinberg (Eds.), *Cognitive processes in writing*. Hillsdale, NJ: Lawrence Erlbaum Associates.

Heaton, P., & Winterston, P. (1996). *Dealing with dyslexia*. London: Whurr.

Henry, M. (1988). Beyond phonics: Integrated decoding and spelling instruction based on word origin and structure. *Annals of Dyslexia, 38*, 258-275.

Hermann, K. (1959). *Reading disability: A medical study of word-blindness and related handicaps*. Copenhagen: Munksgaard.

Hertzig, M., & Farber, E. (1995). *Annual progress in child psychiatry and child development 1994: A selection of the year's outstanding contributions to understanding and treatment of the normal and disturbed child*. New York: Brunner/Mazel.

Hiebert, E. (1994). Reading recovery in the United States: What difference does it make to an age cohert? *Educational Researcher, 23*, 15-25.

Hinshelwood, J. (1917). *Congenital word-blindness*. London: Lewis.

Hogben, J. (1997). How does a visual transient deficit affect reading? In C. Hulme & M. Snowling (Eds.), *Dyslexia: Biology, cognition, and intervention*. London: Whurr.

Hugdahl, K. (1993). Functional brain asymmetry, dyslexia, and immune disorders. In A. Galaburda (Ed.), *Dyslexia and development. Neurobiological aspects of extra-ordinary brains*. Cambridge, MA: Harvard University Press.

Hugdahl, K. (1995). *Psychophysiology: The mind-body perspective*. Cambridge, Mass.: Harvard University Press.

Hulme, C. (1987). Reading retardation. In J. Beech & A. Colley (Eds.), *Cognitive approaches to reading*. Chichester: Wiley.

Humphreys, G., & Bruce, V. (1989). *Visual cognition. Computational, experimental, and neuropsychological perspectives*. Hillsdale, NJ: Lawrence Erlbaum Associates.

Humphreys, G., & Evett, L. (1985). Are there independent lexical and nonlexical routes in word processing? An evaluation of the dual-route theory of reading. *Behavioral and Brain Sciences, 8*, 689-740.

Humphreys, P., Kaufmann, W., & Galaburda, A. (1990). Neuropathological findings in three patients. *Annals of Neurology, 28*, 727-738.

Hurford, D., Johnston, M., Nepote, P., Hamton, S., Moore, S., Neal, J., Mueller, A., McGeorge, K., Huff, L., Awad, A., Tatro, C., Juliano, C., & Huffman, D. (1994). Early identification and remediation of phonological-processing deficits in first-grade children at risk for reading disabilities. *Journal of Learning Disabilities, 27*, 647-659.

Hynd, G. (1997). Dyslexia and gyral morphology variation. In C. Hulme & M. Snowling (Eds.), *Dyslexia: Biology, cognition and intervention*. Cambridge: Whurr.

Hynd, G., Hiémenz, J., Alarcon, M., & Olson, R. (1997). Dyslexia and gyral morphology variation. In C. Hulme & M. Snowling (Eds.), *Dyslexia: Biology, cognition, and intervention*. London: Whurr.

Høien, T. (1979). *Ikonisk persistens og dysleksi*. Stavanger: Rogalandsforskning (doctoral thesis).

Høien, T. (1982). *Ekkoisk persistens og den auditive persepsjonen*. Linköping: Pedagogiska Institutionen, Universitetet i Linköping (doctoral thesis).

Høien, T., & Legaard, O. (1991). Diagnosing word decoding problems - a process-analytical approach. *Reading and Writing: An Interdisciplinary Journal, 3*, 75-89.

Høien, T., & Lundberg, I. (1989a). A strategy for assessing problems in word recognition among dyslexics. *Scandinavian Journal of Educational Research, 33*, 185-201.

Høien, T., & Lundberg, I. (1989b). *KOAS. Kartlegging av ordavkodingsstrategier*. Stavanger: Stiftelsen Dysleksiforsking.

Høien, T., & Lundberg, I. (1989c). *KOAP. Kartlegging av ordavkodingsprosesser*. Stavanger: Stiftelsen Dysleksiforsking.

Høien, T., & Lundberg, I. (1997). *Dysleksi*. Oslo: Ad Notam Gyldendal.

Høien, T., Lundberg, I., Larsen, J., & Tønnessen, F. (1989). Profiles of reading related skills in dyslexic families. *Reading and Writing: An Interdisciplinary Journal, 1*, 381-392.

Høien, T., Lundberg, I., Stanovich, K., & Bjaalid, I.-K. (1995). Components of phonological awareness. *Reading and Writing: An Interdisciplinary Journal, 7*, 1-18.

Iversen, S., & Tunmer, W. (1993). Phonological processing skills and the Reading Recovery program. *Journal of Educational Psychology, 8*, 112-126.

Jacobson, C., & Lundberg, I. (in print). Early prediction of individual growth in reading. *Reading and Writing: An Interdisciplinary Journal.*

Jansen, M. (1989). Tekstens visuelle framtrædelseform. In M. Dalby, C. Elbro, M. Jansen, & T. Krohg (Eds.), *Bogen om læsning II*. København: Munksgaard.

Jarvella, R., Lundberg, I., & Bromley, H. (1989). How immediate is language understanding? Investigating reading in real time. *Reading and Writing. An Interdisciplinary Journal, I*, 103-122.

Johnson, D., & Myklebust, H. (1967). *Learning disabilities. Educational principles and practices.* New York: Grune & Stratton.

Jorm, A., & Share, D. (1983). Phonological recoding and reading acquisition. *Applied Psycholinguistics, 4*, 103-147.

Joshi, M. & Leong, C. (1993). *Reading disabilities: Diagnosis and component processes.* Dordrecht, The Netherlands: Kluwer Academic Publishers.

Joshi, M., Williams, K., & Wood, J. (1998). Predicting reading comprehension from listening comprehension: Is this the answer to the IQ debate? In C. Hulme & M. Joshi (Eds.), *Reading and spelling. Development and disorders*. Mahwah, NJ: Lawrence Erlbaum Associates.

Juel, C. (1988). Learning to read and write: A longitudinal study of 54 children from first through fourth grades. *Journal of Educational Psychology, 80*, 437-447.

Juel, C. (1996). What makes literacy tutoring effective? *Reading Research Quarterly, 31*, 268-289.

Just, M., & Carpenter, P. (1980). A theory of reading: From eye fixation to comprehension. *Psychological Review, 87*, 329-354.

Kao, H., Galen, G., & van Hoosain, R. (1986). *Graphonomics: Contemporary research in handwriting.* Amsterdam: North-Holland.

Karlsdottir, R. (1996a). Print-script as initial handwriting style I: Effects on the development of handwriting. *Scandinavian Journal of Educational Research, 40*, 161-174.

Karlsdottir, R. (1996b). Print-script as initial handwriting style II: Effects on the development of reading and spelling. *Scandinavian Journal of Educational Research, 40*, 255-262.

Karlsdottir, R. (1996c). Development of cursive handwriting. *Perceptual and Motor Skills, 82*, 659-673.

Kavale, K., & Reese, J. (1992). The character of learning disabilities: An Iowa Profile. *Learning Disabilities Quarterly, 15*, 74-94.

Kennedy, A. (1993). Eye movement control and visual display units. In D. Willows, R. Kruk, & E. Corcos (Eds.), *Visual processes in reading and reading disabilities*. Hillsdale, NJ: Lawrence Erlbaum Associates.

Kitz, W., & Tarver, S. (1989). Comparison of dyslexic and nondyslexic adults on decoding and phonemic awareness tasks. *Annals of Dyslexia, 39*, 196-205.

Knivsberg, A. (1997). Urine patterns, peptide levels and IgA/IgG antibodies to food proteins in children with dyslexia. *Pediatric Rehabilitation, I*, 25-33.

Lamb, S., & Gregory, A. (1993). The relationship between music and reading in beginning readers. *Educational Psychology: An International Journal of Experimental Educational Psychology, 13*, 19-27.

Landerl, K., Wimmer, H., & Frith, U. (1997). The impact of orthographic consistency on dyslexia: A German-English comparison. *Cognition, 63*, 315-334.

Larsen, J., Høien, T., Lundberg, I., & Ødegaard, H. (1990). MRI Evaluation of the size and symmetry of the planum temporale in adolescents with developmental dyslexia. *Brain and Laguage, 39*, 289-301.

Larsen, J., Høien, T., & Ødegaard, H. (1992). Magnetic resonance imaging of the corpus callosum in developmental dyslexia. *Cognitive Neuropsychology, 9*, 123-134.

Layton, C., & Koenig, A. (1998). Increasing reading fluency in elementary students with low vision through repeated readings. *Journal of Visual Impairment and Blindness, 92*, 276-293.

Legaard, O. (1987). *Hjerneskader og læsning*. Oslo: Universitetsforlaget.

Leiner, H., Leiner, A., & Dow, R. (1991). The human cerebro-cerebellar systems: Its computing, cognitive, and language skills. *Behavioural Brain Research, 44*, 113-128.

Leiner, H., Leiner, A., & Dow, R. (1993). Cognitive and language functions of the human cerebellum. *Trends in Neuroscience, 16,* 444-447.

Lennerstrand, G., & Ygge, J. (1995). *Visual and occulomotor functions in dyslexia.* Stockholm, Sweden: Department of Ophthalmology, Karolinska Institute.

Levander, S., & Lindgren, M. (1995). *Dyslexi bland intagna på kriminalvårdsanstalten i Malmö.* Malmö.

Levy, C., & Ransdell, S. (1996). *The Science of writing. Theories, methods, individual differences, and applications.* Mahwah, NJ: Lawrence Erlbaum Associates.

Liberman, I., Liberman, A., Mattingly, I., & Shankweiler, D. (1980). Orthography and the beginning reader. In J. Kavanagh & R. Venezky (Eds.), *Orthography, reading and dyslexia.* Baltimore: University Park Press.

Lie, A. (1991). Effects of a training program for stimulating skills in word analysis in first-grade children. *Reading Research Quarterly, 26,* 234-250.

Lie, I. (1989). Visual anomalies, visually related problems and reading difficulties. *Optometrie, 4,* 15-20.

Lindamood, C., & Lindamood, P. (1975). *Auditory discrimination in depth* Chicago, Ill.: Riverside Publishing.

Lindamood, C., Bell, N., & Lindamood, P. (1997). Achieving competence in language and literacy by training in phonemic awareness, concept imagery and comparator function. In C. Hulme & M. Snowling (Eds.), *Dyslexia: Biology, cognition, and intervention.* London: Whurr.

Livingstone, M., Rosen, G., Drislane, F., & Galaburda, A. (1991). Physiological and anatomical evidence for a magnocellular defect in developmental dyslexia. *Proceedings of the National Academy of Science, 88,* 7943-7947.

Locke, J., Hodgson, J., Macaruso, P., Roberts, J., Lambrecht-Smith, S., & Guttentag, C. (1997). The development of developmental dyslexia. In C. Hulme & M. Snowling (Eds.), *Dyslexia: Biology, cognition, and intervention* London: Whurr.

Lovegrove, W., & Williams, M. (1993). Visual temporal processing deficits in specific reading disability. In D. Willows, R. Kruk, & E. Corcos (Eds.), *Visual processes in reading and reading disabilities.* Hillsdale, NJ: Lawrence Erlbaum Associates.

Lovegrove, W., Martin, F., & Slaghuis, W. (1986). A theoretical and experimental case for a visual deficit in specific reading disability. *Cognitive Neuropsychology, 3,* 225-267.

Lubs, H., Duara, R., Levin, B., Jallad, B., Lubs, M., Rabin, M., Kushch, A., & Gross-Glenn, K. (1993). Dyslexia subtypes: Genetics, behavior, and brain imaging. In D. Duane & D. Gray (Eds.), *The reading brain. The biological basis of dyslexia.* Parkton, Maryland: York Press.

Lundberg, I. (1985). Longitudinal studies of reading difficulties in Sweden. In G. MacKinnon & T. Waller (Eds.), *Reading research: Advances in theory and practice. Vol. 4.* New York: Academic Press.

Lundberg, I. (1994). Reading difficulties can be predicted and prevented: A Scandinavian perspective on phonological awareness and reading. In C. Hulme & M. Snowling (Eds.), *Reading development and dyslexia.* London: Whurr.

Lundberg, I., & Høien, T. (1990). Patterns of information processing skills and word recognition in developmental dyslexia. *Scandinavian Journal of Educational Research, 34,* 231-240.

Lundberg, I., & Høien, T. (1997). Levels of approaching reading and its difficulties. In B. Ericson & J. Rönnberg (Eds.), *Reading disability and its treatment* Linköping: Läspedagogiska Institutet EMIR.

Lundberg, I., & Nilsson, L. (1986). What church examination records can tell us about the inheritance of reading disability. *Annals of Dyslexia, 36,* 217-236.

Lundberg, I., & Olofsson, Á. (1993). Can computer speech support reading comprehension. *Computers in Human Behavior, 9,* 283-293.

Lundberg, I., & Tornéus, M. (1978). Nonreaders' awareness of the basic relationship between spoken and written language. *Journal og Experimental Child Psychology, 24,* 404-412.

Lundberg, I., Frost, J., & Petersen, D. (1988). Long term effects of a preschool training program in phonological awareness. *Reading Research Quarterly, 28,* 263-284.

Lundberg, I., Olofsson, Á., & Wall, S. (1980). Reading and spelling skills in the first school years predicted from phonemic awareness skills in kindergarten. *Scandinavian Journal of Psychology, 21,* 159-173.

Lyon, G. (1994). *Frames of reference for the assessment of learning disabilities. New views on measurement issues.* Baltimore, MD: Paul Brookes.

Lyon, G. (1995). Toward a definition of dyslexia. *Annals of Dyslexia, 45,* 3-27.

Lyon, G., & Krasneger, N. (1996). *Attention, memory and executive function.* London: Paul Brookes.

Manis, F., Seidenberg, M., Doi, L., McBride-Chang C., Petersen, A., et al. (1996). On the basis of two subtypes of developmental dyslexia. *Cognition, 58,* 157-195.

Markman, E. (1977). Realization that you don't understand: Elementary school children's awareness of inconsistencies. *Child Development, 50,* 643-655.

Marshall, J., & Newcombe, F. (1973). Patterns of paralexia. *Journal of Psycholinguistic Research, 2,* 175-199.

Martos, F., & Vila, J. (1990). Differences in eye movements control among dyslexic, retarded and normal reader in the Spanish population. *Reading and Writing: An Interdisciplinary Journal, 2,* 175-188.

Masonheimer, P., Drum, P., & Ehri, L. (1984). Does environmental print identification lead children into word reading? *Journal of Reading Behavior, 16,* 257-271.

McConkie, G. (1983). *Eye movements and perception during reading.* New York: Academic Press.

McConkie, G., & Zola, D. (1987). Visual attention during eye fixations while reading. In M. Coltheart (Ed.), *Attention and performance, XII.* London: Lawrence Erlbaum Associates.

McGuinness, D. (1997). *Why our children can't read.* New York: The Free Press.

McLagan, F., Fawcett, A., & Nicolson, R. (1997). *Skill training for dyslexic children: A comparison of different approaches.* Orton Society Conference. Boston.

McLoughlin, D., Fitzgibbon, G., & Young, V. (1994). *Adult dyslexia: Assessment, counselling and training.* London: Whurr.

Mewhort, D., & Campbell, A. (1981). Towards a model of skilled reading: An analysis of performance in tachistoscopic tasks. In G. MacKinnon & T. Waller (Eds.), *Reading research: Advances in theory and practice. Vol. 3.* New York: Academic Press.

Miller Guron, L. (1999). *Wordchains test.* London: NFER Nelson.

Moats, L. (1983). A comparison of the spelling errors of old dyslexic and second-grade normal children. *Annals of Dyslexia, 33,* 121-140.

Moats, L. (1993). Spelling error analysis: Beyond the phonetic/dysphonetic dichotomy. *Annals of Dyslexia, 43,* 174-185.

Moats, L. (1995). *Spelling: Development, disabilities and instruction.* Baltimore: York Press.

Moats, L. (1996). Phonological spelling errors in the writing of dyslexic adolescents. *Reading and Writing: An Interdisciplinary Journal, 8,* 105-119.

Morais, J. (1991). Metaphonological abilities and literacy. In M. Snowling, (Ed.), *Dyslexia: Integrating theory and practice.* London: Whurr.

Morais, J., Cary, L., Algeria, J., & Bertelson, P. (1979). Does awareness of speech as a sequence of phones arise spontaneously? *Cognition, 7,* 323-331.

Morgan, W. (1896). A case of congenital word-blindness. *British Medical Journal, 2,* 1378.

Morris, D. (1992). What constitutes at-risk: Screening children for first grade reading intervention. *School Speech Language Pathology, 2,* 41-51.

Morris, D. (1995). *First Steps: An early reading intervention program.* ERIC Document Reproduction Service No. ED 388 956.

Morris, D., & Perney, J. (1994). Developmental spelling as a predictor of first-grade reading achievement. *The Elementary School Journal, 84,* 441-457.

Morton, J. (1979). Word recognition. In J. Morton & J. Marshall (Eds.), *Psycholinguistic series, Vol. 2.* Cambridge: Mass: MIT Press.

Mosberg, L., & Johns, D. (1994). Reading and listening comprehension in college students with developmental dyslexia. *Learning Disabilities Research & Practice, 9,* 130-135.

National Research Council (1998). *Preventing reading difficulties in young children.* Washington DC: National Academy Press.

Naylor, C., Felton, R., & Wood, F. (1990). Adult outcome in developmental dyslexia. In G. Pavlidis (Ed.), *Perspectives on dyslexia. Vol. 2: Cognition, language and treatment.* New York: Wiley.

Newman, A., Lewis, W., & Beverstock, C. (1994). *Prison Literacy: Implications for program and assessment.* University of Pennsylvania: National Center on Adult Literacy.

Nicolson, R., & Fawcett, A. (1994a). Comparison of deficits in cognitive and motor skills among children with dyslexia. *Annals of Dyslexia, 44,* 147-164.

Nicolson, R., & Fawcett, A. (1994b). Comparison of deficit severity across skills: Towards a taxonomy for dyslexia. In A. Fawcett & R. Nicolson (Eds.), *Dyslexia in Children. Multidisciplinary Perspectives.* London: Harvester Wheatsheaf.

Nicolson, R., Fawcett, A., Berry, E., Jenkins, I., Dean, P., & Brooks, D. (in print). *Cerebellar function is impaired in dyslexia: A PET activation study.*

Niemi, P., Kinnunen, R., Poskiparta, E., & Vauras, M. (1999). Do pre-school data predict resistance to treatment in phonological awareness, decoding and spelling? In I. Lundberg, F. Tønnessen, & I. Austad (Eds.), *Dyslexia: Advances in theory and practice.* Dordrecht, NL: Kluwer Academic Publishers.

Oakhill, J., Cain, K., & Yuill, N. (1998). Individual differences in children's comprehension skills: Toward an integrated model. In C. Hulme & M. Joshi (Eds.), *Reading and spelling. Development and disorders* Mahwah, NJ: Lawrence Erlbaum Associates.

Oakhill, J., & Yuill, N. (1996). Higher order factors in comprehension disability: Processes and remediation. In C. Cornoldi & J. Oakhill (Eds.), *Reading comprehension difficulties. Processes and intervention.* Mahwah, NJ: Lawrence Erlbaum Associates.

Obrzut, J., & Hynd, G. (1991). *Neuropsychological foundations of learning disabilities. A handbook of issues, methods, and practice.* New York: Academic Press.

O'Connor, N., & Hermelin, B. (1994). Two autistic savant readers. *Journal of Autism and Developmental Disorders, 24,* 501-515.

Oftedal, M., & Høien, T. (1997). *KOAP. Håndbok. Et program for kartlegging av ordavkodingsprosesser.* Stavanger: Stiftelsen Dysleksiforsking.

Olofsson, Å., & Lundberg, I. (1985). Evaluation of long term effects of phonemic awareness training in kindergarten. Illustration of some methodological problems in evaluation research. *Scandinavian Journal of Psychology, 26,* 21-34.

Olson, R., & Forsberg, H. (1993). Disabled and normal readers' eye movements in reading and nonreading tasks. In D. Willows, R. Kruk, & E. Corcos (Eds.), *Visual processes in reading and reading disabilities.* Hillsdale, NJ: Lawrence Erlbaum Associates.

Olson, R., Forsberg, H., Wise, B., & Rack, J. (1994). Measurement of word recognition, orthographic, and phonological skills. In G. Lyon (Ed.), *Frames of reference for the assessment of learning disabilities.* Baltimore: Paul Brookes.

Olson, R., Wise, B., Conners, F., & Rack, J. (1989). Organization, heritability, and remediation of component word recognition and language skills in disabled readers. In T. Carr & B. Levy (Eds.), *Reading and its development: Component skills approaches.* New York: Academic Press.

Olson, R., Wise, B., Johnson, M., & Ring, J. (1997). The etiology and remediation of phonologically based word recognition and spelling disabilities: Are phonological deficits the "hole" story? In B. Blachman (Ed.), *Foundations of reading acquisition and dyslexia. Implications for early intervention.* London: Lawrence Erlbaum Associates.

Orton Dyslexia Society. (1997). *Informed instruction for reading success: Foundations for teacher preparation.* The Orton Dyslexia Society.

Orton, S. (1937). *Reading, writing and speech problems in children.* London: Chapman & Hall.

Owen, F. (1978). Dyslexia - Genetic aspects. In A. Benton & D. Pearl (Eds.), *Dyslexia: An appraisal of current knowledge.* New York: Oxford University Press.

Palinscar, A., & Brown, A. (1985). Reciprocal teaching: A means to a meaningful end. In J. Osborn, P. Wilson, & R. Anderson (Eds.), *Reading education: Foundations for a literate America.* Lexington, Ma.: D.C. Heath.

Paulesu, E., Frith, U., Snowling, M., Gallagher, A., Morton, J., Frackowiak, R., & Frith, C. (1996). Is developmental dyslexia a disconnection syndrome? Evidence from PET scanning. *Brain, 119,* 143-157.

Pavlidis, G. (1981). Sequencing, eye movements and the early objective diagnosis of dyslexia. In G. Pavlidis & T. Miles (Eds.), *Dyslexia research and its applications to education.* New York: Wiley.

Pavlidis, G. (1991a). Do eye movements hold the key to dyslexia. *Neuropsychologia, 19,* 57-64.

Pavlidis, G. (1991b). Diagnostic significance and relationship between dyslexia and erratic eye movements. In J. Stein (Ed.), *Vision and visual dyslexia.* London: MacMillan.

Pearson, P., & Leys, M. (1985). Teaching comprehension. In T. Harris & E. Cooper (Eds.), *Reading, thinking and concept development*. New York: College Board Publications.

Pennington, B. (1991). *Reading disabilities: Genetic and neurological influences*. London: Kluwer Academic Publishers.

Pennington, B. (1997). Using genetics to dissect cognition. *American Journal of Human Genetic, 60*, 13-16.

Pennington, B., Groisser, D., & Welsh, M. (1993). Contrasting cognitive deficits in attention deficit hyperactivity disorder versus reading disability. *Child Development, 29*, 511-523.

Pennington, B., McCabe, L., Smith, S., Lefly, D., Bookman, M., Kimberling, W., & Lubs, H. (1986). Spelling errors in adults with a form of familial dyslexia. *Child Development, 57*, 1001-1013.

Pennington, B., van Orden, G., Smith, S., Green, P., & Haith, M. (1990). Phonological processing skills and deficits in adult dyslexics. *Child Development, 61*, 1753-1778.

Perfetti, C. (1969). Lexical density and phrase structure depth as variables in sentence retention. *Journal of Verbal Learning and Learning Behavior, 8*, 719-724.

Peterson, M., & Haines, L. (1992). Orthographic analogy training with kindergarten children: Effects on analogy use, phonemic segmentation, and letter-sound knowledge. *Journal of Reading Behavior, 24*, 109-127.

Pinnell, G., Huck, C., DeFord, D., Bryk, A., & Seltzer, A. (1994). Comparing instructional models for the literacy education of high-risk first graders. *Reading Research Quarterly, 29*, 9-38.

Pirozzolo, F., & Rayner, K. (1978). The neural control of eye movements in acquired developmental reading disorders. In H. Avakian-Whitaker & H. Whitaker (Eds.), *Advances in neurolinguistics and psycholinguistics*. New York: Academic Press.

Pollatsek, A. (1993). Eye movements in reading. In D. Willows, R. Kruk, & E. Corcos (Eds.), *Visual processes in reading and reading disabilities*. Hillsdale, NJ: Lawrence Erlbaum Associates.

Poskiparta, E., Vauras, M., & Niemi, P. (1998). Promting word recognition, spelling and reading comprehension skills in a computer-based training program in grade 2. In P. Reitsma & L. Verhoeven (Eds.), *Problems and interventions in literacy development*. Dordrecht, NL: Kluwer Academic Publishers.

Postlethwaite, N., & Ross, K. (1992). *Effective schools in reading. Implications for educational planners*. Hamburg: The International Association for the Evaluation of Educational Achievement.

Pramling, I. (1988). *Att lära barn att lära*. Göteborg: Universitetet i Göteborg.

Pressley, M., Rankin, J., & Yokoi, L. (1996). A survey of instructional practices of outstanding primary-level literacy teachers. *Elementary School Journal, 96*, 363-384.

Pressley, M. et al. (1989). Memory strategy research in learning disabilities: Present and future. *Learning Disabilities Research, 4*, 68-72.

Rack, J., Hulme, C., Snowling, M., & Wightman, J. (1994). The role of phonology in young children learning to read words: The direct mapping hypothesis. *Journal of Experimental Child Psychology, 57*, 42-71.

Raichle, M. (1994). Images of the mind: Studies with modem imaging techniques. *Annual Review of Psychology, 45*, 330-356.

Rankin, J., & Pressley, M. (in print). A survey of instructional practices of primary-grade special education teachers nominated as effective in promoting literacy. *Elementary School Journal*.

Rayner, K. (1990). Comprehension processes: Introduction. In D. Balota, G. Flores d'Arcais, & K. Rayner (Eds.), *Comprehension processes in reading*. Hillsdale, NJ: Lawrence Erlbaum Associates.

Rayner, K. (1997). Understanding eye movements in learning to read. *Scientific Studies of Reading, 1*, 317-339.

Read, C. (1978). Children's awareness of language, with emphasis on sound systems. In A. Sinclair, R. Jarvella, & W. Levelt (Eds.), *The child's conception of language*. New York: Springer-Verlag.

Read, C. (1996). *Children's creative spelling*. London: Routledge and Kegan Paul.

Reid, G. (1995). Toward a definition of dyslexia. *Annals of Dyslexia, 45*, 3-27.

Reiff, H. et al., (1992). Learning to achieve: Suggestions from adults with learning disabilities. *Journal of Postsecondary Education and Disability, 10*, 11-22.

Reiff, H., Gerber, P., & Gensberg, R. (1994). Instructional strategies for long-term success. *Annals of Dyslexia, 1994*, 270-288.

Riccio, C., & Hynd, G. (1996). Neuroanatomical and neurophysiological aspects of dyslexia. *Topics in Language Disorders, 16,* 1-13.

Rice, M. (1996). *Toward a genetics of language.* Mahwah, NJ: Lawrence Erlbaum Associates.

Riddoch, M., & Humphreys, G. (1983). The effects of cueing on unilateral neglect. *Neuropsychologia, 21,* 589-599.

Rispens, J. (1990). Comprehension problems in dyslexia. In D. Balota, G. Flores d'Arcais, & K. Rayner (Eds.), *Comprehension processes in reading.* Hillsdale, NJ: Lawrence Erlbaum Associates.

Rosen, G., Sherman, G., & Galaburda, A. (1991). Interhemispheric connections differ between symmetrical and asymmetrical brain regions. *Neuroscience, 41,* 779-790.

Rosen, G., Sherman, G., & Galaburda, A. (1993). Dyslexia and brain pathology: Experimental animal models. In A. Galaburda (Ed.), *Dyslexia and development. Neurobiological aspects of extra-ordinary brains.* Cambridge, MA: Harvard University Press.

Runyon, M. (1991). The effect of extra time on reading comprehension scores for university students with and without learning disabilities. *Journal of Learning Disabilities, 2,* 104-107.

Samuels, J. (1985). Automaticity and repeated reading. In P. Osborn, R. Wilson, & R. Anderson (Eds.), *Reading education: Foundations for a literate America.* Lexington: Lexington Press.

Samuelsson, S., Gustavsson, A., Herkner, B., & Lundberg, I. (in print). Is the frequency of dyslexic problems among prison inmates higher than in a normal population? *Reading and Writing: An Interdisciplinary Journal.*

Santa, C. (1995). *Content reading including study systems. Reading, writing and studying across the curriculum.* Iowa: Kendal/Hunt Publishing Company.

Santa, C., & Høien, T. (1999). An assessment of Early Steps: A program for early intervention of reading problems. *Reading Research Quarterly, 34,* 54-79.

Scanlon, D., & Vellutino, F. (1997). Instructional influences on early reading success. *Perspectives. The International Dyslexia Association, 23,* 35-37.

Scarborough, H. (1984). Continuity between childhood and adult reading. *British Journal of Psychology, 75,* 329-348.

Scarborough, H. (1990). Very early language deficits in dyslexic children. *Child Development, 61,* 1728-1743.

Schupack, H., & Wilson, B. (1997). *Reading. writing and spelling. The multisensory structured language approach.* Baltimore: The International Dyslexia Association.

Schrott, L., Denenberg, V., Sherman, G., Waters, N., Rosen, G., & Galaburda, A. (1992). Environmental enrichment neocortical ectopias, and behavior in the autoimmune NZB mouse. *Developmental Brain Research, 67,* 85-93.

Searls, E. (1985). *How to use WISC-R scores in reading/learning disability diagnosis.* Newark: International Reading Association.

Seidenberg, M., & McClelland, J. (1989). A distributed, developmental model of word recognition and naming. *Psychological Review, 96,* 523-568.

Seymour, P. (1990). Developmental dyslexia. In M. Eysenck (Ed.), *Cognitive psychology: An international review.* Chichester, England: Wiley.

Seymour, P., & Elder, L. (1992). Beginning reading without phonology. *Cognitive Neuropsychology, 3,* 1-36.

Seymour, P., & Evans, H. (1992). Beginning reading without semantics: A cognitive study of hyperlexia. *Cognitive Neuropsychology, 9,* 889-122.

Seymour, P., & Evans, H. (1994). Levels of phonological awareness and learning to read. *Reading and Writing: An Interdisciplinary Journal, 6,* 221-250.

Seymour, P., & Porpodas, C. (1980). Lexical and non-lexical processing of spelling in dyslexia. In U. Frith (Ed.), *Cognitive processes in spelling.* London: Academic Press.

Shallice, T. (1981). Phonological agraphia and the lexical route in writing. *Brain, 104,* 413-429.

Shallice, T., & Warrington, E. (1980). Single and multiple component central dyslexic syndromes. In M. Coltheart, K. Patterson, & J. Marshall (Eds.), *Deep dyslexia.* London: Routledge & Kegan Paul.

Share, D., & Stanovich, K. (1995). Has the phonologial recoding model of reading acquisition and reading disabilitiy led us astray? *Issues in Education, 1,* 1-57.

Shaywitz, B., et al. (1996). The functional organization of brain for reading and reading disability (Dyslexia). *The Neuroscientist, 2,* 245-255.

Shuren, J., Maher, L., & Heilman, K. (1996). The role of visual imagery in spelling. *Brain and Language, 52,* 365-372.

Siegel, L. (1992). An evaluation of the discrepancy definition of dyslexia. *Journal of Learning Disabilities, 25,* 619-629.

Siegel, L. (1993). The development of reading. *Advances in child development and behavior, 24,* 63-97.

Siegel, L. (1994). Phonological processing deficits as the basis of developmental dyslexia: Implications for remediation. In M. Riddhoch & G. Humphreys (Eds.), *Cognitive neuropsychology and cognitive rehabilitation.* Hillsdale, NJ.: Lawrence Erlbaum Associates.

Siegel, L., Geva, E., & Share, D. (1992). The development of orthographic skills in normal and disabled readers. *Psychological Science, 6,* 250-254.

Simpson, S., Sawnson, J., & Kunkel, K. (1992). The impact of an intensive multisensory reading program on a population of learning disabled delinquents. *Annals of Dyslexia, 42,* 54-66.

Skaalvik, S. (1994). *Voksne med lese- og skrivevansker forteller om sine skoleerfaringer* (doctoral thesis). Trondheim: Norsk Voksenpedagogisk Forskningsinstitutt.

Skjelfjord, V. (1977). *Metoden i den første leseundervisningen .* Oslo: Gyldendal Norsk Forlag.

Smith, F. (1973). *Psycholinguistics and reading.* New York: Holt, Rinehart, & Winston.

Smith, S., Kimberling, W., & Pennington, B. (1991). Screening for multiple genes influencing dyslexia. In B. Pennington (Ed.), *Reading disabilities: Genetic and neurological influences.* London: Kluwer Academic Publishers.

Smith, S., Kimberling, W., Pennington, B., & Lubs, H. (1983). Specific reading disability: Identification of an inherited form through linkage analysis. *Science, 219,* 1345-1347.

Snowling, M. (1981). Phonemic deficits in developmental dyslexia. *Psychological Research, 43,* 219-234.

Snowling, M., & Nation, K. (1997). Language, phonology, and learning to read. In C. Hulme & M. Snowling (Eds.), *Dyslexia: Biology, cognition, and intervention.* London: Whurr.

Spafford, C., & Grosser, G. (1996). *Dyslexia: Research and resource guide.* Boston: Reading Literacy in the United States.

Spear-Swerling, L., & Sternberg, R. (1994). The road not taken: An integrative theoretical model of reading disability. *Journal of Learning Disabilities, 27,* 91-104.

Spear-Swerling, L., & Sternberg, R. (1996). *Off track. When poor readers become "learning disabled".* Boulder, CO: Westview Press.

Spedding, S., & Chan, L. (1993). Metacognition, word identification, and reading competence. *Contemporary Educational Psychology, 18,* 91-100.

Spiegel, D. (1995). A comparison of traditional remedial programs and Reading Recovery: Guidelines for success for all programs. *The Reading Teacher, 49,* 86-96.

Stanovich, K. (1986). Matthew effects in reading: Some consequences of individual differences in the acquisition of literacy. *Reading Research Quarterly, 21,* 360-407.

Stanovich, K. (1988). The right and wrong places to look at for the cognitive locus of reading disabilities. *Annals of Dyslexia, 38,* 154-177.

Stanovich, K. (1991). Discrepancy definitions of reading disability: Has intelligence led us astray? *Reading Research Quarterly, 26,* 7-29.

Stanovich, K. (1996). The role of inadequate print exposure as a determinant of reading comprehension problems. In C. Cornoldi & J. Oakhill (Eds.), *Reading comprehension difficulties: Processes and intervention.* Hillsdale, NJ: Lawrence Erlbaum Associates.

Stanovich, K., & Siegel, L. (1994). The phenotypic performance profile of reading disabled children: A regression-based test of the phonological-core variable-difference model. *Journal of Educational Psychology, 86,* 24-53.

Stanovich, K., Siegel, L., & Gottardo, A. (1997a). Converging evidence for the phonological and surface subtypes of reading disability. *Journal of Educational Psychology, 89,* 114-127.

Stanovich, K., Siegel, L., & Gottardo, A. (1997b). Progress in the search for dyslexia sub-types. In C. Hulme & M. Snowling (Eds.), *Dyslexia: Biology, cognition, and intervention.* London: Whurr.

Stanovich, K., Siegel, L., Gottardo, A., Chiappe, P., & Sidhu, R. (1997c). Subtypes of developmental dyslexia: Differences in phonological and orthographic coding. In B. Blachman (Ed.), *Foundations of reading acquisition and dyslexia.* London: Lawrence Erlbaum Associates.

Stein, J. (1993). Visuospatial perception in disabled readers. In D. Willows, R. Kruk, & E. Corcos (Eds.), *Visual processes in reading and reading disabilities.* Hillsdale, NJ: Lawrence Erlbaum Associates.

Stein, J., & Fowler, M. (1982). Diagnosis of dyslexia by means of a new indicator of eye dominance. *British Journal of Ophthalmology, 66,* 332-336.

Stein, J., & Fowler, M. (1985). Effect of monocular occlusion on visuomotor perception and reading in dyslexic children. *The Lancet, 2,* 69-73.

Stein, J., & Walsh, V. (1997). To see but no to read: The magnocellular theory of dyslexia. *The Trends in Neuroscience, 20,* 147-152.

Stein, J., Riddle, P., & Fowler, M. (1988). Disordered vergence eye movement control in dyslexic children. *British Journal of Ophtalmology, 712,* 162-166.

Stevenson, J., Graham, P., Fredman, G., & McLoughlin, V. (1986). A twin study of genetic influences on reading and spelling ability and disability. *Journal of Child Psychology and Psychiatry, 28,* 231-247.

Söderbergh, R. (1971). *Reading in early childhood: A linguistic study of a preschool child's gradual acquisition of reading ability.* Stockholm: Almquist & Wiksell.

Søvik, N., & Arntzen, O. (1992). Different tracking techniques in training graphic behaviour of "normal" and dysgraphic children. *European Journal of Special Needs Education, 7,* 156-168.

Søvik, N., Arntzen, O., & Karlsdottir, R. (1993). Relations between writing speed and some other parameters in handwriting. *Journal of Human Movement Studies, 25,* 133-150.

Søvik, N., Arntzen, O., & Samuelstuen, M. (1993). A study of the relations between process and product variables in writing. In G. Eigler & T. Jechle (Eds.), *Writing, current trends in European research.* Freiburg: Hochschul Verlag.

Søvik, N., Heggberget, M., & Samuelstuen, M. (1996). Strategy-training related to children's text production. *British Journal of Educational Psychology, 66,* 169-180.

Søvik, N., Samuelsson, M., Svara, K., & Lie, A. (1996). The relationship between linguistic characteristics and reading/writing performance of Norwegian children. *Reading and Writing: An Interdisciplinary Journal, 8,* 199-216.

Tallal, P. (1980). Auditory temporal perception, phonics and reading disabilities in children. *Brain and Language, 9,* 182-198.

Tallal, P., Miller, S., & Fitch, R. (1993). Neurobiological basis of speech: A case for preminence of temporal processing. *Annals of the New York Academy of Science, 682,* 27-48.

Taube, K. (1988). *Reading acquisition and self-concept.* Umeå: University of Umeå.

Taylor, I., & Taylor, M. (1983). *The psychology of reading.* New York: Academic Press.

Topping, K., & Parkinson, E. (1996). Paired reading, spelling and writing: The handbook for teachers and parents. *Child Language Teaching and Therapy, 12,* 354-357.

Torgesen, J., Morgan, S., & Davis, C. (1992). The effects of two types of phonological awareness training on word learning in kindergarten children. *Journal of Educational Psychology, 84,* 364-370.

Torgesen, J., Wagner, R., & Rashotte, C. (1997). Approaches to the prevention and remediation of phonologically based reading disabilities. In B. Blachman (Ed.), *Foundations of reading and dyslexia. Implications for early intervention.* London: Lawrence Erlbaum Associates.

Treiman, R. (1992). The role of intrasyllabic units in learning to read and spell. In P. Gough, L. Ehri, & R. Treiman (Eds.), *Reading acquisition.* Hillsdale, NJ: Lawrence Erlbaum Associates.

Treiman, R. (1993). *Beginning to spell: A study of first grade children.* New York: Oxford University Press.

Treiman, R. (1997). Spelling in normal readers and dyslexics. In B. Blachman (Ed.), *Foundations of reading acquisition and dyslexia. Implications for early intervention.* Mahwah, NJ: Lawrence Erlbaum Associates.

Tuley, A. (1998). *Never too late to read. Language skills for adolescent with dyslexia.* Baltimore: York Press.

Tønnesen, G. (1995). *Lesevansker og atferdsvansker. Teoretiske studier og en empirisk undersøkelse.* Stavanger: Høgskolen i Stavanger.

Tønnessen, F. (1995). *Leselyst og lesestoff.* Stavanger: Senter for leseforsking.

Tønnessen, F., Løkken, A., Høien, T., & Lundberg, I. (1993). Dyslexia, left-handedness, and immune disorders. *Archives of Neurology, 50,* 411-416.

Vellutino, F., & Scanlon, D. (1989). Some prerequisite for interpreting results from reading level matched designs. *Journal of Reading Behavior, 21,* 361-385.

Vellutino, F., Scanlon, D., & Tanzman, M. (1994). Components of reading ability. Issues and problems in operationalizing word identification, phonological coding, and orthographic coding. In G. Lyon (Ed.), *Frames of reference for the assessment of learning disabilities* Baltimore: Paul Brookes.

Vellutino, F., Scanlon, D., & Sipay, E. (1997). Towards distinguishing between cognitive and experimental deficits as primary sources of early intervention in diagnosing specific reading disabilities. In B. Blachman (Ed.), *Foundations of reading and dyslexia. Implications for early intervention.* London: Lawrence Erlbaum Associates.

Vellutino, F., Scanlon, D., Sipay, E., Small, S., Pratt, A., Chen, R., & Denckla, M. (1996). Cognitive profiles of difficulty-to-remediate and readily remediated poor readers: Early identification as a vehicle for distinguishing between cognitive and experimental deficits as basic causes of specific reading disability. *Journal of Educational Psychology, 88,* 601-638.

Vernon, M. (1957). *Backwardness in reading.* Cambridge: Cambridge University Press.

Wagner, R., Torgesen, J., & Rashotte, C. (1994). Development of reading-related phonological processing abilities: Evidence of bi-directional causality from latent variable longitudinal study. *Developmental Psychology, 30,* 73-87.

Wasik, H., & Slavin, R. (1993). Preventing early reading failure with one-to-one tutoring: A review of five programs. *Reading Reseach Quarterly, 28,* 179-200.

Weisberg, P. (1988). Direct instruction in the preschool. *Educational and Treatment of Children, 11,* 249-363.

West, T. (1992). A future of reversals: Dyslexic talents in a world of computer visualization. *Annals of Dyslexia, 42,* 124-139.

White, W. (1992). The postschool adjustment or persons with learning disabilities: Current status and future projections. *Journal of Learning Disabilities, 25,* 448-456.

Wiggen, G. (1990). Språksosiologiske aspekt ved rettskrivingsavvik hos norske barneskoleelever. In C. Elbro, C. Liberg, E. Magnusson, K. Naucler, & G. Wiggen (Eds.), *Læsning og skrivning i sprogvidenskabeligt perspektiv.* København: Dafolo Forlag.

Wiggen, G. (1992). *Rettskrivingsstudier 2. Kvalitativ og kvantitativ analyse av rettskrivingsavvik hos østnorske barneskoleelever.* Bd. 1-2. Oslo: Novus forlag.

Willows, D., Kruk, R., & Corcos, E. (1993). *Visual processes in reading and reading disabilities.* Hillsdale, NJ: Lawrence Erlbaum Associates.

Wimmer, H., Mayringer, H., & Landerl, K. (1998). Poor reading: A deficit in skill-automatization or a phonological deficit? *Scientific Studies of Reading, 2,* 321-340.

Wimmer, H., Mayringer, H., & Raberger, T. (1999). Reading and dual-task balancing: Evidence against the automatization deficit explanation of developmental dyslexia. *Journal of Learning Disabilities, 32,* 473-478.

Wise, B., Olson, R., & Ring, J. (1997). Teaching phonological awareness with and without the computer. In C. Hulme & M. Snowling (Eds.), *Dyslexia: Biology, cognition, and intervention.* London: Whurr.

Wise, B., Olson, R., & Treiman, R. (1990). Subsyllabic units in computerized reading instruction: Onset-rime vs postvowel segmentation. *Journal of Experimental Child Psychology, 49,* No. 1.

Wolf, M. (1984). Naming, reading and dyslexias: A longitudinal study. *Annals of Dyslexia, 34,* 87-115.

Wolf, M., & Segal, B. (1992). Word finding and reading in the developmental dyslexias. *Topics in Language Disorders, 13,* 51-65.

Wood, F. (1989). *Brain structure and dyslexia.* Orton Dyslexia Society Meeting. Tampa, Florida.

Worthy, M., & Invernizzi, M. (1990). Spelling errors of normal and disabled students on achievemement levels one through four: Instructional implications. *Annals of Dyslexia, 40,* 138-151.

Worthy, J., & Vise, N. (1996). Morphological, phonological, and orthographic differences between the spelling of normally achieving children and basic literacy adults. *Reading and Writing: An Interdisciplinary Journal, 8,* 139-159.

Yap, R., & van der Leij, A. (1994a). Automaticity deficits in word reading. In A. Fawcett & R. Nicolson (Eds.), *Dyslexia in children. Multidisciplinary perspectives.* London: Harvester Wheatsheaf.

Yap, R., & van der Leij, A. (1994b). Testing the automatization deficit hypothesis of dyslexia via a dual-route paradigm. *Journal of Learning Disabilities, 27,* 660-665.

AUTHOR INDEX

SUBJECT INDEX

NEUROPSYCHOLOGY AND COGNITION

The purpose of the Neuropsychology and Cognition series is to bring out volumes that promote understanding in topics relating brain and behavior. It is intended for use by both clinicians and research scientists in the fields of neuropsychology, cognitive psychology, psycholinguistics, speech and hearing, as well as education. Examples of topics to be covered in the series would relate to memory, language acquisition and breakdown, reading, attention, developing and aging brain. By addressing the theoretical, empirical, and applied aspects of brain-behavior relationships, this series will try to present the information in the fields of neuropsychology and cognition in a coherent manner.

1. P.G. Aaron: *Dyslexia and Hyperlexia.* 1989
   ISBN 1-55608-079-4; 1994, Pb 0-7923-3155-9
2. R.M. Joshi (ed.): *Written Language Disorders.* 1991   ISBN 0-7923-0902-2
3. A. Caramazza: *Issues in Reading, Writing and Speaking.* A Neuropsychological Perspective. 1991   ISBN 0-7923-0996-0
4. B.F. Pennington (ed.): *Reading Disabilities.* Genetic and Neurological Influences. 1991   ISBN 0-7923-1606-1
5. N.H. Hadley: *Elective Mutism.* A Handbook for Educators, Counsellors and Health Care Professionals. 1994   ISBN 0-7923-2418-8
6. W.C. Watt (ed.): *Writing Systems and Cognition.* Perspectives from Psychology, Physiology, Linguistics, and Semiotics. 1994   ISBN 0-7923-2592-3
7. I. Taylor and D.R. Olson (eds.), *Scripts and Literacy.* Reading and Learning to Read Alphabets, Syllabaries and Characters. 1994   ISBN 0-7923-2912-0
8. V.W. Berninger (ed.): *The Varieties of Orthographic Knowledge.* I: Theoretical and Developmental Issues. 1994   ISBN 0-7923-3080-3
9. C.K. Leong and R.M. Joshi (eds.): *Developmental and Acquired Dyslexia.* Neuropsychological and Neurolinguistic Perspectives. 1995
   ISBN 0-7923-3166-4
10. N. Gregg: *Written Expression Disorders.* 1995   ISBN 0-7923-3355-1
11. V.W. Berninger (ed.): *The Varieties of Orthographic Knowledge.* II: Relationships to Phonology, Reading, and Writing. 1995   ISBN 0-7923-3641-0
    Set (Vols 8 + 11) ISBN 0-7923-3081-1
12. Y. Lebrun (ed.): *From the Brain to the Mouth.* Acquired Dysarthria and Dysfluency in Adults. 1997   ISBN 0-7923-4427-8
13. J. Rispens, T.A. van Yperen and W. Yule (eds.), *Perspectives on the Classification of Specific Developmental Disorders.* 1998   ISBN 0-7923-4871-0
14. C.K. Leong and K. Tamaoka (eds.), *Cognitive Processing of the Chinese and the Japanese Languages.* 1998   ISBN 0-7923-5479-6
15. P. Reitsma and L. Verhoeven (eds.), *Problems and Interventions in Literacy Development.* 1998   ISBN 0-7923-5557-1

NEUROPSYCHOLOGY AND COGNITION

16. I. Lundberg, F.E. Tønnessen and I. Austad (eds.): *Dyslexia: Advances in Theory and Practice*. 1999   ISBN 0-7923-5837-6
17. T. Nunes (ed.), *Learning to Read: An Integrated View from Research and Practice*. 1999   ISBN 0-7923-5513-X
18. T. Høien and J. Lundberg: *Dyslexia: from Theory to Intervention*. 2000
ISBN 0-7923-6309-4

KLUWER ACADEMIC PUBLISHERS – DORDRECHT / BOSTON / LONDON

Printed in the United Kingdom
by Lightning Source UK Ltd.
130154UK00001B/262/A